An Outline of Swine Diseases

A HANDBOOK

AN OUTLINE OF
Swine Diseases

A HANDBOOK

Ross P. Cowart, DVM, MS

IOWA STATE UNIVERSITY PRESS / AMES

Ross P. Cowart, DVM, is Associate Professor of Food Animal Medicine and Surgery in the College of Veterinary Medicine, University of Missouri–Columbia. He is a Diplomate of the American Board of Veterinary Practitioners in the Food Animal Practice Specialty.

♾ Printed on acid-free paper in the United States of America

First edition, 1995

Library of Congress Cataloging-in-Publication Data

Cowart, Ross P.
An outline of swine diseases: a handbook/Ross P. Cowart.—1st ed.
p. cm.
Includes index.
ISBN 0-8138-2899-6
1. Swine—Diseases—Handbooks, manuals, etc. I. Title.
SF971.C695 1995
636.4′089—dc20 95-22163

CONTENTS

Preface vii

1. Swine Production Medicine **3**
The Veterinarian's Role in Swine Production 3
Swine Health and Management 4
Pathogen avoidance 5
Pathogen elimination 6
Management of the environment 8
Immunizations 10
Medications 15

2. Polysystemic Diseases **23**
Erysipelas 23
Glasser's Disease 25
Porcine Reproductive and Respiratory Syndrome (PRRS) 26
Pseudorabies 28
Salmonellosis 32

3. Respiratory Diseases **35**
Atrophic Rhinitis 35
Inclusion Body Rhinitis 40
Necrotic Rhinitis 41
Swine Influenza 41
Pulmonary Bordetellosis 43
Mycoplasmal Polyserositis 44
Pleuropneumonia 45
Mycoplasmal Pneumonia 48
Pasteurellosis 50
Verminous Pneumonia 51

4. Gastrointestinal Diseases **54**
Colibacillosis 54
Transmissible Gastroenteritis (TGE) 56
Rotaviral Enteritis 59

Coccidiosis 60
Clostridial Enteritis 62
Postweaning Scours 64
Swine Dysentery 66
Proliferative Enteropathy 70
Hemorrhagic Bowel Syndrome 71
Whipworms 72
Gastric Ulcers 73

5. Central Nervous System Diseases 75
Myoclonia Congenita 75
Neonatal Hypoglycemia 76
Streptococcal Meningitis 77
Salt Poisoning 79
Edema Disease 80

6. Musculoskeletal Diseases 82
Neonatal Polyarthritis 82
Splay-Leg 83
Suppurative Arthritis 84
Mycoplasmal Arthritis 85
Rickets 87
Foot Lesions 88
Osteochondrosis 89
Osteomalacia 91
Porcine Stress Syndrome (PSS) 92

7. Reproductive and Urogenital Diseases 94
Porcine Parvovirus (PPV) 94
Leptospirosis 96
Postparturient Dysgalactia 97
Vulvar Discharge 100
Cystitis/Pyelonephritis 103
Seasonal Infertility 105

8. Integumentary Diseases 106
Mange 106
Lice 108
Exudative Epidermitis 108
Swine Pox 110

9. Circulatory Diseases 111
Mulberry Heart Disease 111
Baby Piglet Anemia 112
Eperythrozoonosis 113

Index 115

Preface

This document is, as the title suggests, an *outline* of swine diseases. It is intended to provide the reader with some basic facts about swine medicine in a concise outline format. My original purpose for producing this outline was to supplement a series of swine medicine lectures that I deliver to veterinary students each year. Although there are excellent textbooks that deal with swine diseases, my students need a more concise summary of some of the more important information regarding swine medicine, especially considering the limited time they have to study this subject. This outline has evolved to fill that need.

I also discovered that some practicing veterinarians (who are not primarily swine specialists) have found this outline useful in their occasional encounters with pigs. It has been used as a review guide for licensing and specialty board exams. I believe that this outline could also serve as an effective client-education tool for swine specialty practitioners. The positive comments I have received from students and practitioners have motivated me to make this outline available to a larger audience.

The outline begins with comments on the veterinarian's role in swine production and a discussion of swine health management techniques. I believe that this section is a very important part of the text, for it reflects the swine industry's realization that we must, by economic necessity, shift emphasis from treatment and management of disease to health maintenance. The disease sections are organized by the body system affected. Some diseases that have major effects on several body systems have been grouped in a section on polysystemic diseases. The systems approach allows the reader to consider as a group those diseases that may show similar clinical signs.

This outline is not intended as a comprehensive reference work; a conscious decision has been made to sacrifice completeness for brevity. Diseases that are uncommon or absent from the United States are not presented, and diseases of nutritional or toxic origin are given only limited coverage. I urge those who need a more complete and detailed text to avail themselves of the excellent references that exist. I suggest:

Leman, AD, et al., eds. *Diseases of Swine*. Seventh Edition. Ames: Iowa State University Press, 1992.
This is unquestionably the best reference text on swine diseases. I highly recommend that any serious scholar of swine medicine obtain this book.

Taylor, DJ. *Pig Diseases*. Fifth Edition. Cambridge, England: The Burlington Press, 1989.
This is a readable and affordable book, written from the British perspective. Some of the terminology and disease conditions are different in the United Kingdom, but not enough to limit the usefulness of this book.

Howard, JL, ed. *Current Veterinary Therapy: Food Animal Practice 3*. Philadelphia: W.B. Saunders Co., 1993.
This book covers other food animal species and is not exhaustive in its coverage of swine diseases, but some of the chapters on swine diseases are excellent.

Blood, DC, and Radostits, OM. *Veterinary Medicine*. Seventh Edition. London: Baillière Tindall, 1989.
This is a good general food animal and equine text.

Many textbooks are out of date soon after publication. The swine practitioner needs timely information in the rapidly changing field of swine medicine, and one of the best ways to keep up is to join the American Association of Swine Practitioners (AASP). In addition to the information this organization provides via its annual meeting, the AASP supplies its membership with a subscription to the journal *Swine Health and Production*, proceedings of other major swine medicine meetings (including the biannual International Pig Veterinary Society Congress), and subscriptions to swine producer journals. Membership dues are reasonable, especially for students. I urge anyone interested in swine medicine to consider the benefits of membership and contact the AASP at 5921 Fleur Drive, Des Moines, Iowa 50321, (515) 285-7808.

I am obliged to many former and present students and colleagues for their assistance in the preparation of this outline and their suggestions for improvement. I owe a debt of gratitude to my mentor, Dr. Lennart Backstrom, who challenged me to learn and offered me a chance to teach. My colleagues at the University of Missouri, especially Drs. Rick Tubbs, Laurie Wallace, Bob Miller, David Weaver, Bill Wolff, and Rick Marion, provided thoughtful discussions, gave large doses of encouragement, and did my other work for me while I prepared this book. Special thanks go to Dr. Tom Gillespie of Rensselaer, Indiana, who, as a practicing swine veterinarian, took the time to critique this outline and to offer many constructive suggestions. The reviewers and editors at Iowa State University Press have been extremely helpful and thoughtful in their criticism. My wife, Diane, has been supportive and patient, tolerating my long hours and blank stares from behind the word-processing screen. Much of what is good about this book can be credited to others, and I would appreciate knowing your suggestions or comments. With your help, future editions will be better than this one.

Ross P. Cowart	voice:	(314) 882-7821
A308 Clydesdale Hall	fax:	(314) 884-5444
379 East Campus Drive	e-mail:	cowart@vth.vetmed.missouri.edu
Columbia, Missouri 65211		

An Outline of Swine Diseases

A HANDBOOK

1

SWINE PRODUCTION MEDICINE

THE VETERINARIAN'S ROLE IN SWINE PRODUCTION

Swine practitioners have several responsibilities in their service to swine production units. Effective practitioners must balance their responsibilities to the producer, the consumer, the animals, and the swine industry as a whole.

A. The veterinarian must effectively serve the swine producer.
   1. The producer's goal is to produce pork profitably.
   2. The ultimate reason for the producer to seek advice from a veterinarian is to maximize profits and/or minimize losses. Therefore, the economic impact of every recommendation we make *must* be carefully considered. For example, the decision to use a particular vaccine or drug must be evaluated in terms of costs (materials, labor, professional fee) and of what the anticipated benefits will be (decreased death loss, improved weight gains and feed efficiency). To justify a recommendation, the economic returns must be greater than the costs.

B. As an advisor to an industry that is providing food for humans, the veterinarian must also be concerned about the quality and wholesomeness of the final product of that industry.
   1. The consumer expects pork bought at the grocery store to be palatable and of high quality.
   2. Most consumers have limited knowledge of modern animal agricultural methods, nevertheless, they expect the food they buy to be free of chemicals or drugs that may have been used in the production of that food.
   3. The veterinarian's influence should be used to assure that any animal under his or her care goes into the food supply free of chemotherapeutic residues. Indeed, a veterinarian can be held liable for a residue resulting from treatments performed or advised by him or her, particularly if the treatments were not precisely as directed on the label.

C. The veterinarian must also be concerned about the animal itself.
   1. We dedicate ourselves to the "relief of animal suffering" when we speak the veterinarians' oath. The maintenance of animal health is obviously in the animal's best interest.
   2. However, maximal animal health is not always consistent with maximal profits.
      a. For example, repair of a fractured femur in a feeder pig may be in the animal's best interest but is seldom cost effective. Few would argue against the humane destruction of this animal.
      b. A more difficult example is the case of an overcrowded finishing barn, which can produce a greater overall profit than one that is not overcrowded even though the performance (average daily gain, feed efficiency) of each individual pig is less in the overcrowded barn.
   3. The whole subject of animal welfare is full of emotion and relatively devoid of facts. Fortunately, the facts are becoming known as research into issues of animal welfare becomes more common. The veterinarian should become familiar with the available facts.
   4. Changes in production practices for the sake of animal welfare are probably necessary and inevitable. These changes, however, should be based on what is truly best for the animal rather than on poorly informed, totally emotional responses.

D. At times, veterinarians must look beyond their responsibilities to individual producers and consider their responsibilities to the swine industry as a whole.
   1. Many times, a veterinarian is called upon to participate in government animal disease control programs. Usually this takes the form of examining and testing animals for sale or show for certain reportable diseases (e.g., pseudorabies, brucellosis).
   2. The success of such animal disease control programs depends on the responsibility and integrity of the practicing veterinarian.

SWINE HEALTH AND MANAGEMENT

There is little doubt that the interests of swine producers and their animals are better served by the maintenance of health than by the treatment of disease. Health is defined in *Dorland's* as "a state of optimal physical, mental, and social well-being, and not merely the absence of disease and infirmity." Therefore, animal health is inextricably linked to animal welfare. Since swine production is an enterprise intended to bring profit to the producer, we should expand the above definition to include "a state of optimal economic productivity."

Management is a broad term referring to the interaction of people and animals and is an essential determinant of swine health and productivity. In modern swine production, the manager takes responsibility for providing a healthy physical and social environment and adequate nutrition for the animals. In return, we expect the animals to convert a lower value product (feed) into a higher value product (pork). In this section, we examine some techniques that managers can use to maximize health, production, and economic return.

A. Management techniques for pathogen avoidance
   1. Some organisms are serious primary pathogens, and our goal should be to eliminate them from the herd if present and to avoid them altogether if absent. Examples of these diseases include pseudorabies, brucellosis, swine dysentery, and transmissible gastroenteritis (TGE). Avoidance of these causative pathogens is accomplished primarily by:
      a. Isolating and testing incoming animals before they are introduced to the rest of the herd.
      b. Controlling the access of possible fomites, or carriers, e.g., people, pets, birds, wildlife.
   2. Most swine diseases are caused by endemic and opportunistic pathogens. These diseases usually occur when the pathogen population in the environment is great enough to overcome the animal's resistance or when some other stressor decreases the animal's resistance. Such diseases include colibacillosis, salmonellosis, rotaviral enteritis, streptococcal meningitis, Glasser's disease, and pasteurellosis. Techniques for avoiding the pathogens of these diseases include:
      a. Sanitation. Cleaning and disinfection of pens between groups and regular removal of manure from pens can go a long way toward controlling many diseases. Thorough cleaning is the most important step in sanitation. All organic matter should be washed away. Power washers that spray hot water under high pressure are needed for thorough cleaning.
      b. All-in, all-out rearing. Most diseases are transmitted from older carrier animals to younger susceptible animals. If pigs are farrowed in groups and moved through the production system as a group without being mixed with other groups, many disease problems can be avoided.
         i. For all-in, all-out production to work properly, careful scheduling and proper facility design is critical. For example, let us assume that a producer is farrowing a group of sows every 3 weeks. Sows should be bred to farrow within a narrow time range, preferably 7 days or less. Pigs will all be weaned on the same day and moved as a group to the nursery facility. Sows will also be moved to the breeding facility that same day. The empty farrowing room will be thoroughly cleaned and disinfected before the next group enters. Pigs will be moved through the production facilities (e.g., nursery, grower, finisher) as a group, and each facility will be cleaned and disinfected between groups. Each nursery, grower, and

finisher facility should be designed to handle the same number of pigs.

ii. Research and experience indicates that all-in, all-out production improves both daily gain and feed efficiency 7% to 10%.

iii. Many producers will run the farrowing house and nursery on an all-in, all-out basis while the grower/finisher facilities are continuous flow. Although this is better than nothing, recognize that the majority of the economic benefits of all-in, all-out rearing are realized during the grower/finisher stages of production.

iv. A variation on all-in, all-out production that is gaining popularity is *multiple site production*. The principles are the same as all-in, all-out, however, the farrowing, nursery, and grower/finisher facilities are each at different geographic sites. This reduces the chances of airborne transmission of pathogens between buildings on the same site.

B. Management techniques for pathogen elimination. Swine producers are realizing that some diseases are simply too costly to live with. Several methods have evolved to eliminate these diseases from a herd. Herds established by one of these methods are sometimes called *minimal disease herds*.

1. SPF (specific-pathogen-free) program

a. The SPF program is based on the concept that, most of the time, pigs get pathogenic organisms from other pigs. The normal pig is basically germ-free before birth. Its first exposure to potential pathogens occurs during birth (vaginal flora) and shortly after birth (exposure to the dam). Therefore, if the pig is delivered by caesarean section and raised in isolation from other pigs (including its dam), it should be free of most pathogenic organisms. Certain SPF laboratories are certified to derive these pigs, which, therefore, are sometimes called Lab pigs.

b. Primary SPF herds are established with Lab pigs. Herd additions must be either from the Lab, artificial insemination, or embryo transfer.

c. Secondary SPF herds are established from primary herds. Herd additions must be from primary herds, artificial insemination, embryo transfer, or the Lab.

d. All SPF herds are monitored for and certified free of turbinate atrophy, pneumonic lesions, swine dysentery, lice, mange, TGE, and pseudorabies.

e. SPF herds can be a good source of healthy animals for starting or repopulating a commercial herd.

f. SPF pigs may not be the best source of replacement animals for herds with a high level of disease problems. Because of their minimal disease status, the immune system of SPF pigs is naive to many swine pathogens. SPF pigs often become quite ill when introduced into high-disease herds.

2. Segregated (Medicated) early weaning (SEW, MEW)
    a. Segregated early weaning was developed as a way to eliminate or decrease certain diseases without the expense, trouble, and loss of genetic material associated with depopulation and repopulation with SPF stock.
    b. The original concept of medicated early weaning was developed by Alexander et al. in the United Kingdom. It was based on the assumption that it takes several weeks for the neonatal pig to acquire the microflora of an adult pig. It also assumed that the biggest piglets in the litter had consumed the most colostrum and thus were more resistant to disease. In the original procedure:
        i. Pregnant sows were removed from the source herd in late gestation and placed in an isolated farrowing facility.
        ii. Sows were induced to farrow on the same day.
        iii. The largest piglets were weaned at 5 days of age and moved to an isolated nursery unit.
        iv. Sows and piglets were given prophylactic antibiotic treatments.
        v. Infection with *Mycoplasma hyopneumoniae*, *Bordetella bronchiseptica*, and colonic spirochetes was eliminated or significantly reduced in MEW pigs compared to conventionally reared pigs.
    c. Harris modified Alexander's original method to allow for later weaning (10-20 days) and farrowing sows at the source farm. Sows are immunized with several antigens prior to farrowing to enhance colostral immunity. Weaned pigs are still moved to an isolated nursery unit. Age segregation and isolation appear to be more important factors than medication in disease control. SEW pigs consistently outperform their conventionally raised counterparts.
3. Depopulation/Repopulation (depop/repop)
    a. Many times, the quickest and simplest way to get rid of a disease problem is to get rid of the pigs. Repopulation should be from minimal disease herds (e.g., SPF, SEW).
    b. There are two potential liabilities associated with depop/repop: loss of genetic material and nonproductive downtime.
        i. Loss of genetic material usually concerns only the seedstock producer. Many commercial producers could improve their genetic base by depop/repop.
        ii. Since all animals at a site must be removed for a depopulation, there is a period of nonproductive downtime. However, most high- disease herds make up for the downtime with improved productivity and lower treatment costs within a year or two after repopulation.

C. Management of the environment

1. Thermal environment

   a. Swine are susceptible to stress from either heat or cold. Temperature can have a profound effect on behavior, energy balance, feed intake, and resistance to disease. Several terms are useful in our discussion of the thermal environment:

      i. Effective environmental temperature is determined by the actual air temperature plus other factors that may make the environment feel warmer or cooler. For example, moisture and drafts decrease the effective environmental temperature; straw bedding (insulation) increases the effective environmental temperature. Floor surfaces can also influence effective environmental temperature, e.g., wood is warmer than concrete, which is warmer than woven wire.

      ii. Thermoneutral zone is the range of effective environmental temperatures in which the animal's heat production is roughly equivalent to heat losses. No special heat conserving or heat dissipating mechanisms are needed. Just below the thermoneutral zone is the *cool zone*, in which the animal must invoke physiological mechanisms to conserve heat (e.g., peripheral vasoconstriction, piloerection). Just above the thermoneutral zone is the *warm zone*, in which the animal must invoke physiological mechanisms to dissipate heat (e.g., vasodilation). As the temperature rises, the animal reduces its activities in an attempt to decrease metabolic heat production.

      iii. Lower critical temperature is the effective environmental temperature below which an animal must increase its metabolic rate to maintain body heat. Energy is diverted from normal metabolic processes to maintaining body temperature. This animal is experiencing cold stress.

      iv. Upper critical temperature is the effective environmental temperature at which heat-dissipating mechanisms are at maximal effectiveness. Above this temperature, the animal cannot maintain normal body temperature.

   b. Temperatures at which thermal stress occurs vary with the size of the animal and with the stage of production.

      i. Neonatal pigs are especially susceptible to cold stress. Their lower critical temperature may be as high as 88°F (31°C). The lower critical temperature for a finishing pig on full feed is 57°F (14°C).

      ii. Lactating sows are especially susceptible to heat stress. Sows that are too hot usually reduce their feed intake, and may not consume enough calories to sustain lactation.

      iii. Wide fluctuations in temperature may be more stressful than high or low absolute temperatures. Variation in temperature over a 24-hour period should not exceed 15°-20°F (8°-11°C), and changes should be gradual over the 24 hours. High/low thermometers may be useful in monitoring temperature fluctuations. Automatic and/or frequent adjustments of side curtains and air inlets may be necessary during times of rapidly changing weather.

2. Air environment
   a. Noxious gases
      i. Ammonia is formed from the decomposition of urine and feces. Higher levels of ammonia are produced when excreta collects on a solid floor (especially with straw bedding) than when it is deposited into a liquid slurry pit below a slatted or wire floor. Ammonia is the most common noxious gas found in swine buildings. It irritates the mucous membranes of the eye and respiratory tract. This can decrease growth performance and increase susceptibility to respiratory infections.
      ii. Hydrogen sulfide is probably the most dangerous noxious gas found in swine buildings. It is formed from the decomposition of excreta in an anaerobic pit. Normally the concentration of hydrogen sulfide in swine buildings is less than 10 ppm and is not toxic at this level. However, when a pit is agitated in preparation for being pumped out, levels can rapidly rise to 1000 ppm or greater. Pigs and humans exposed to this level die within minutes. Buildings should be emptied and well ventilated before the pit is agitated. If you detect the characteristic "rotten egg" odor of hydrogen sulfide, **leave the building immediately!**
      iii. Carbon monoxide is formed from the incomplete combustion of fuel. This occurs most commonly in swine buildings when a gas heater is improperly adjusted and improperly vented to the outside. Carbon monoxide competes with oxygen for binding sites on hemoglobin, resulting in hypoxia. Fetal hemoglobin has a greater affinity for carbon monoxide than does adult hemoglobin. A common clinical history for carbon monoxide intoxication is a high incidence of stillbirths in a farrowing house in the winter.
   b. Dust
      i. Large dust particles (10-15 μm) irritate the upper airway.
      ii. Small dust particles (1-3 μm) irritate the lower airway.
      iii. Dried fecal dust (endotoxin) and animal dander (allergen) are probably the most significant respiratory irritants. Feed dust is probably more of a nuisance than a health threat.
3. Social environment
   a. Group size. Most nursery, grower, and finisher pigs are housed in groups. There is some evidence that the optimal group size is

roughly the size of one litter (8 to 10 pigs). Dominance orders are more stable in litter-sized groups than in larger groups. However, pigs have been kept in groups as large as 50 with no apparent adverse effects.

b. Space requirements. Estimates of space requirements for different size pigs are presented below. Space requirements increase in warm conditions and decrease in cool conditions.

13-20 lb pigs — 1.5-2.0 ft^2/pig
20-50 lb pigs — 2.5-3.0 ft^2/pig
50-100 lb pigs — 4.5-5.0 ft^2/pig
100-240 lb pigs — 6.0-8.0 ft^2/pig

c. Overcrowding undermines the dominance order. Overcrowded pigs are more prone to aggression and behavioral vices, such as tail biting, ear biting, etc.

d. Sorting and mixing pigs should be minimized. Every time a new group is formed, a certain amount of fighting will occur until a new dominance order is established. This diverts the pig's energy away from productive activities (i.e., eating) and increases the probability of injury.

D. Immunizations

1. Vaccines are merely tools we can use in the attempt to tip the scales in favor of animal health. Vaccines are not perfect, and vaccination does not always result in immunization. Vaccines may fail to provide protection for a variety of reasons, including improper handling and administration. Sometimes vaccines fail simply because the challenge dose of the pathogenic organism overcomes the immunity provided by the vaccine. We should avoid thinking that since we have vaccinated for a certain disease that the animals are absolutely "immune" to the disease.

2. A decision to vaccinate for a certain disease should be based on real or perceived economic benefit. The costs of vaccination (including costs for materials and labor) should be less than the benefits derived from vaccination (e.g., decreased death losses, improved rate of gain and feed efficiency, increased reproductive efficiency, etc.). The risk of not vaccinating should also be assessed. Risk assessment should consider the history of disease on the farm, the incidence of disease in the area, and herd security. The efficacy of the vaccine and potential side effects should also be considered.

3. With few exceptions, vaccines should be used in accordance with label directions. Timing of vaccination will vary depending on the target of immune response. For example, if the target of protection is the neonatal pig then the dam should be vaccinated prefarrowing (usually 5 weeks and/or 2 weeks prior to farrowing) to stimulate colostral antibodies for passive transfer. If the target of protection is the young nursery or grower

pig, each individual pig should be vaccinated (may be given preweaning or postweaning, depending on the product) to stimulate active immunity. If the vaccine is intended to protect breeding animals from reproductive diseases, it is usually given shortly prior to breeding.

4. Below is a partial list of antigens that are available in swine vaccines. Many variations and combinations are produced (222 vaccines are listed in the 1992 *Compendium of Swine Products*). Most products contain one or more of the following antigens:
   a. Erysipelas
      i. Killed bacterins and modified live vaccines are available.
      ii. Vaccination is generally effective in preventing acute, fatal septicemic disease. It may not provide total protection against chronic joint and heart disease.
      iii. Prevalence of asymptomatic infection is fairly high. Most herds contain carriers; therefore, risk of exposure is high. Most herds that are not vaccinated will eventually experience losses from erysipelas. Vaccine is relatively inexpensive. Routine vaccination is probably a cost-effective procedure in most herds.
      iv. Vaccination is usually done first at or shortly after weaning, and again in 3-5 weeks. Breeding animals are vaccinated every 6 months.
   b. Leptospirosis
      i. Killed bacterins containing up to 6 serovars of lepto are available.
      ii. Vaccination will reduce but not eliminate reproductive losses from leptospirosis.
      iii. Subclinical infections are common. Risk of exposure is high. Routine vaccination is commonly recommended.
      iv. Vaccination is usually first given at 6-7 months of age (prior to first breeding) and every 6 months thereafter (i.e., prior to subsequent breedings).
   c. Parvovirus
      i. Killed virus vaccines are available.
      ii. Prevalence of infection is high. Practically 100% of unvaccinated swine will become infected between 6 and 12 months of age. Natural infection confers a solid immunity that probably lasts a lifetime.
      iii. Vaccination provides some immunity (although less than natural infection), which probably lasts 4 to 6 months.
      iv. Vaccination is usually first given at 6-7 months of age and every 6 months thereafter (same as lepto, in fact, lepto and parvo are often combined in a single product).
   d. Bordetella/Pasteurella (atrophic rhinitis [AR])
      i. Most of these vaccines are killed bacterins. A modified live

intranasal Bordetella vaccine is available. Some of the bacterins include a Pasteurella toxoid.

ii. Infection is common, although some minimal disease herds may be free of *Bordetella* and *Pasteurella*. Not every herd that is infected experiences significant economic losses from AR. Vaccination should be reserved for those herds that are experiencing significant losses from AR.

iii. Vaccination schedule varies with different products. Most suggest vaccination of the sow once or twice prefarrowing to stimulate colostral antibodies, and vaccination of the piglets to stimulate active immunity.

iv. Currently *Pasteurella multocida* toxin is thought to be a primary factor in severe, growth retarding AR. Therefore, if vaccination is indicated, the vaccine used should contain toxigenic strains of *Pasteurella multocida* and a toxoid as well.

e. *Escherichia coli*

i. Commercial vaccines are usually killed whole cell bacterins or pilus subunit vaccines. Some include an enterotoxin toxoid.

ii. Infection with enterotoxigenic *E. coli* is common. However, many herds experience no significant losses from colibacillosis, especially if management and sanitation is good. Vaccination is difficult to justify in herds with a history of minimal problems with neonatal pig diarrhea.

iii. Vaccine is given to gilts twice prefarrowing and sows once or twice prefarrowing to stimulate colostral immunity.

iv. Commercial vaccines are usually fairly efficacious against most of the enteropathogenic serotypes of *E. coli*. In problem herds, autogenous bacterins or the Kohler milk vaccine may be helpful.

f. Transmissible gastroenteritis (TGE)

i. Modified live virus oral vaccine and killed virus injectable vaccines are available.

ii. Risk of exposure is high in some herds. Herds in areas of high swine population density and herds with poor security against exposure to wildlife and birds are at greater risk. Herds in isolated areas with good security measures are at lower risk.

iii. Vaccines are better at eliciting an anamnestic response from a natural infection than at eliciting a primary response, therefore, TGE vaccination works better against endemic, chronic TGE than against acute TGE.

iv. Vaccine is given to sows and gilts prefarrowing to stimulate colostral immunity. A reduced oral dose may be given to neonatal piglets.

v. Controlled exposure of sows and gilts to virulent virus by feeding them minced intestines from neonates that have died from TGE probably induces the best immunity. Without careful management and sanitation, this also has the danger of perpetuating the virus in the environment.

g. Rotavirus
   i. Modified live virus and killed virus vaccines are available.
   ii. Virus is ubiquitous, therefore risk of exposure is high; however many well-managed herds have little problem with rotavirus diarrhea.
   iii. In problem herds, vaccine may be given to the sow pre-farrowing and/or the piglets preweaning.

h. *Clostridium perfringens* type C
   i. Killed bacterins, toxoids, and antitoxins are available.
   ii. Infection is relatively uncommon; however, some herds and some areas of the country have a high level of infection and significant losses. Vaccination can be useful in problem herds.
   iii. Usually bacterins and toxoids are given to the sow pre-farrowing and the antitoxin is given to piglets shortly after birth.

i. Swine dysentery (*Serpulina [Treponema] hyodysenteriae*)
   i. Vaccine is a killed whole cell bacterin.
   ii. Although many herds are infected, it is difficult to cost effectively live with the disease. The best means of control is avoidance of infection or elimination of infection if present.
   iii. Vaccine may reduce clinical signs, but will not prevent infection or the development of a carrier state.
   iv. If used, vaccine should be given first at 6 to 8 weeks of age and repeated in 3 weeks. Boosters may be given at other times when disease breaks are anticipated.

j. *Actinobacillus (Haemophilus)* pleuropneumonia
   i. Available vaccines are killed bacterins.
   ii. Vaccination is more effective in preventing acute death losses than it is in preventing chronic pleuropneumonia. The disease can still be costly even in vaccinated herds.
   iii. Vaccine is given to pigs at or shortly after weaning and again 3-4 weeks later.

k. Glasser's disease (*Haemophilus parasuis*)
   i. A killed whole cell bacterin is available.
   ii. Although infection is common, the disease is subclinical in most herds. Minimal disease herds seem to be the most susceptible to outbreaks of clinical Glasser's disease. Use of vaccine in these herds may be cost effective.
   iii. Vaccine is given to pigs at or shortly after weaning and again 3-4 weeks later.

l. *Streptococcus suis*

i. Bacterins and antisera are available.
ii. Infection is more common than clinical disease. Stress may precipitate outbreaks.
iii. If used, vaccine is given at or shortly after weaning and again in 2-3 weeks. Antiserum is given before the anticipated onset of disease.

m. Salmonellosis
i. Killed whole cell bacterins have been available for some time. These have been limited in efficacy. A *Salmonella* vaccine has been produced that stimulates the production of anti-endotoxin antibodies. Modified live *Salmonella* vaccines have recently been approved and show some promise. The cost effectiveness of any of these products is unknown and should be evaluated on each farm.
ii. Vaccination is usually done at or around weaning time and again 2-3 weeks later or just before disease typically breaks.

n. *Mycoplasma hyopneumoniae*
i. Killed bacterins have recently been introduced.
ii. The economic impact of disease should be established before vaccination can be recommended. The vaccine may reduce lesions and improve growth rates in some herds.
iii. The recommended time of vaccination varies with product. Most call for two doses preweaning.

o. Encephalomyocarditis (EMC) virus
i. A killed virus vaccine is available.
ii. The vaccine is indicated as an aid in the prevention of reproductive failure in gilts and sows and in the prevention of economic losses in pigs caused by infection with encephalomyocarditis virus. There is no consensus on how frequently this occurs.
iii. Sows and gilts are vaccinated twice prior to breeding.

p. Pseudorabies
i. Modified live and killed virus vaccines are available. Many have antigenic markers that allow differentiation of vaccine titers and natural infection titers.
ii. Pseudorabies vaccination is usually quite effective in suppressing clinical signs of disease.
iii. Pseudorabies vaccination is regulated by state authorities in most states.
iv. If indicated, vaccine is given to pigs at or around weaning and every 6 months thereafter.

q. Swine influenza
i. A killed virus vaccine is available.
ii. Vaccination is reported to decrease clinical signs and reduce virus shedding in challenged pigs.

E. Medications (See Tables 1.1, 1.2, and 1.3 at the end of this chapter.)

1. Our objectives when administering antibacterial drugs to swine generally fall into one of three categories:
   a. Treatment of disease. Antibacterial drugs are indicated for many bacterial infections of swine. For effective treatment of disease, we need to provide a high level of drug (at least a minimum inhibitory concentration) in the infected tissue. With few exceptions, this can be achieved only by parenteral administration of antibacterial drugs.
   b. Prevention or control of disease. Lower levels of antimicrobial drugs are effective in preventing or suppressing disease if given before the animals are ill. Addition of drug to the feed or water of swine can be effective in controlling many diseases.
   c. Improvement in growth rate and feed efficiency. Many drugs can improve the growth rate and feed efficiency of swine when added at very low levels in the feed. The mechanism of this action is not entirely understood.
2. While there are obvious benefits to drug use in swine, the negative aspects must be recognized.
   a. Possibility of residues in meat. If a drug is appreciably absorbed into an animal's blood stream, then residues may be found in meat after the animal is slaughtered. The USDA Food Safety and Inspection Service establishes tolerance levels for many drugs and chemicals, which it believes would represent no health risks to humans consuming that meat. If levels are found beyond the tolerance level, the meat is not passed for human consumption and the reason behind the violative level is investigated.
   b. Negative image to consumers and general public. Many consumers view drug treatments in food animals as something that is unnatural and possibly dangerous. Consumers usually react positively to the idea of food that is "all natural" and contains "no additives."
   c. Development of microbial resistance. Low level antimicrobial use in animal feeds results in an increase in antimicrobial-resistant bacteria in an animal's system. This may make it more difficult to treat disease in the animals and some people believe that it represents a health risk to humans.
3. Strategies of drug use. As mentioned earlier, our objectives are to produce pork cost effectively, protect consumer interests, and promote animal welfare. Unfortunately, these objectives may conflict with one another in decisions regarding drug use in animals.
   a. Drug use in the clinically ill animal. In general, we would like to administer high levels of drugs for a sufficient time to effect a cure. Generally, this involves parenteral injections.
      i. Legally, we may use only approved drugs for the indications listed on the label and at the dosage listed on the label. Frequently, we encounter conditions that cannot be success-

fully treated by an approved drug used according to label directions.

ii. The FDA recognizes that the use of approved drugs according to label directions is inadequate for many diseases. Therefore, as a matter of policy, the FDA will not take enforcement action against the extra-label use of an injectable drug, provided the following conditions are met:
   1) A valid veterinarian/client/patient relationship must exist. The veterinarian must be personally familiar with the condition of the animals, either from a recent examination or from regular visits to the herd.
   2) The veterinarian must determine that an approved drug used according to label directions would not be effective against an animal's condition.
   3) Animals treated with an extra-label drug must be identified and records kept of their treatment. Extended withdrawal times must be observed. The veterinarian will be liable if a violative residue is found.
   4) Under no circumstances may a veterinarian or producer use a drug that has been declared illegal for use in food-producing animals. Drugs currently listed as illegal include diethylstilbestrol, chloramphenicol, dimetridazole, ipronidazole, nitrofurazone, furazolidone, and clenbuterol.
   5) Drugs administered through the feed may not be used other than as the label directs.

b. Drug use in the clinically normal animal. In general, we would like to administer the smallest amount of drug that will cost effectively achieve our goal of disease prevention or growth promotion.

i. Ideally, drugs used for treatment or prevention of disease should not be used at lower levels for growth promotion. If this is done, bacterial resistance is likely to occur, and the drug will not be as efficacious against the disease if used at the higher level.

ii. Ideally, drugs used for growth promotion should be used only for that purpose, i.e., they should not be used for treatment or prevention of disease. For public health concerns, it is probably best not to use drugs that have application in human medicine for growth promotion in animals.

iii. Many producers and veterinarians tend to classify drugs as *therapeutic drugs* or *production drugs* according to the criteria listed above.

iv. Some veterinarians suggest rotating therapeutic and production drugs through the grower/finisher stage. This allows for the prevention of disease while reducing the likelihood of bacterial resistance.

c. Residue avoidance.

i. In many cases, the avoidance of residues in meat is simply a matter of following directions. Always allow the full withdrawal time period to pass after the last treatment before presenting an animal to slaughter. Longer withdrawal times may be necessary if the drug is used at above label dosages.

ii. Although any drug may cause a residue if used improperly, sulfamethazine has been responsible for more residues than any other drug used in swine. Some of the reasons for these residues include:

1) Failure to follow directions regarding withdrawal time.
2) Carryover in feed handling equipment. If a small amount of medicated feed is left in the mixer when a supposedly "clean" batch of feed is being mixed, the resulting feed may have enough drug contamination to cause a violative residue.
3) Recycling of drug through manure and urine.

iii. The veterinarian can play a very important role in residue avoidance. A number of test kits are available for testing blood or urine of prospective market hogs for drug residues. The National Pork Producers Council (NPPC) sponsors a "Pork Quality Assurance" program that encourages veterinary input into drug-use decisions.

Suggested Reading:

Alexander TJL, Thornton K, Boon G, Lysons RJ, Gush AF. 1980. Medicated early weaning to obtain pigs free from pathogens endemic in the herd of origin. *Vet Rec* 106:114-119.

Harris DL. 1988. Alternative approaches to eliminating endemic diseases and improving performance of pigs. *Vet Rec* 123:422-423

Table 1.1. Drugs used in swine feeds

Name of drug	Trade name (manufacturer)	Use level	With-drawal	Indications
Apramycin	Apralan (Elanco)	150 g/ton for 14 days	28 days	Colibacillosis (weanling pig scours)
Bacitracin methylene disalicylate	BMD (A.L.Labs)	10-30 g/ton	0	Increase rate of gain and feed efficiency
		250 g/ton		Control of swine dysentery Control of clostridial enteritis in suckling pigs (feed to sows from 14 days before to 21 days after farrowing)
Bamber-mycins	Flavomycin (Hoechst)	2-4 g/ton	0	Increase rate of gain and feed efficiency
Carbadox	Mecadox (Pfizer)	10-25 g/ton	10 weeks; do not feed to pigs over 75 lb body wt	Increase rate of gain and feed efficiency
		50 g/ton		Control of swine dysentery Control of bacterial swine enteritis (salmonellosis)
Chlortetracy-cline	Aureomycin (Cyan-amid) PfiChlor (Pfizer) CtC (Fermenta)	10-50 g/ton	0	Increase rate of gain and feed efficiency
		50-100 g/ton		Prevention of bacterial swine enteritis Maintain weight gain in the presence of AR Reduce the incidence of cervical abscesses
		100-200 g/ton		Treatment of bacterial swine enteritis
		200 g/ton		Aid in reducing the spread of leptospirosis
		400 g/ton for 14 days		Aid in reducing shedding of leptospirae Aid in reducing the abortion rate of swine and the mortality rate of newborn pigs when leptospirosis is present
Chlortetracy-cline, sulfa-methazine, penicillin	Aureo S-P 250 (Cyanamid) PhiChlor-250 (Pfizer)	100 g/ton 100 g/ton 50 g/ton	15 days	Reduction of the incidence of cervi-cal abscesses Treatment of bacterial swine enteri-tis (salmonellosis) Maintain weight gain in the pres-ence of AR Increase rate of gain and feed effi-ciency up to 75 lb

Table 1.1. Drugs used in swine feeds (continued)

Name of drug	Trade name (manufacturer)	Use level	With-drawal	Indications
Chlortetracycline, sulfathiazole, penicillin	CSP 250 (Fermenta)	100 g/ton 100 g/ton 50 g/ton	7 days	Reduction of the incidence of cervical abscesses Treatment of bacterial swine enteritis (salmonellosis) Maintain weight gain in the presence of AR Increase rate of gain and feed efficiency up to 75 lb
Lincomycin	Lincomix (TUCO-Upjohn)	20 g/ton	0	Increase rate of gain
		40 g/ton		For control of swine dysentery
		100 g/ton for 3 weeks followed by 40 g/ton	6 days	For treatment and control of swine dysentery
		200 g/ton for 21 days		For reduction in the severity of mycoplasmal pneumonia
Neomycin, oxytetracycline	Neo-Terramycin (Pfizer) NEO/OXTC (Smith-Kline)	35-140 g/ton 50-150 g/ton	10 days if neomycin level is 140 g/ton; 5 days if lower level	As an aid in the prevention (50 g OTC) or treatment (100 g OTC) of bacterial enteritis, baby pig diarrhea, vibrionic dysentery, bloody dysentery, and salmonellosis Maintain weight gains and feed consumption in the presence of AR
Oxytetracycline	Terramycin (Pfizer) OXTC (Smith-Kline)	7.5-10 g/ton	0	Increase rate of gain and feed efficiency
		50 g/ton		As an aid in the prevention of bacterial enteritis, baby pig diarrhea, vibrionic dysentery, bloody dysentery, and salmonellosis
		100 g/ton		As an aid in the treatment of bacterial enteritis, baby pig diarrhea, vibrionic dysentery, bloody dysentery, and salmonellosis
		50 - 150 g/ton		Maintain weight gains and feed consumption in the presence of AR
		500 g/ton for 7 to 14 days	5 days	In the presence of leptospirosis, reduces instances of abortion, gives higher survival rate, heavier and healthier newborn pigs Reduces urinary shedding of leptospirae and aids in maintenance of normal weight gains and feed consumption

Table 1.1. Drugs used in swine feeds (continued)

Name of drug	Trade name (manufacturer)	Use level	With-drawal	Indications
Penicillin	Penicillin P-100 (Pfizer)	10-50 g/ton	0	Aid in stimulating growth and improving feed efficiency
Tiamulin	Denagard (Fermenta)	10 g/ton	0	Increased rate of gain and feed efficiency
		35 g/ton	2 days	Control of swine dysentery
Tylosin	Tylan (Elanco)	10-100 g/ton	0	Increased rate of gain and improved efficiency
		100 g/ton for 3 weeks, then 40 g/ton to market		Prevention of swine dysentery Prevention of proliferative enteritis[a]
		100 g/ton		Maintain weight gain and feed efficiency in the presence of AR
Tylosin, sulfamethazine	Tylan-Sulfa (Elanco)	100 g/ton	15 days	Maintain weight gain and feed efficiency in the presence of AR; lower incidence and severity of *Bordetella bronchiseptica* rhinitis; prevention of swine dysentery; control of pneumonias caused by bacterial pathogens (*P. multocida* and/or *C. pyogenes*)
Virginiamycin	Stafac (SmithKline)	5-10 g/ton	0	Increased rate of gain and improved feed efficiency
		25 g/ton		As an aid in the control of swine dysentery (up to 120 lb)[b]
		100 g/ton for 2 weeks, then 50 g/ton		For treatment and control of swine dysentery (up to 120 lb)[b]

Source: From 1994 Feed Additive Compendium, The Miller Publishing Company, Minnetonka, Minnesota

[a] An unapproved indication but some evidence for efficacy

[b] A label claim, but not generally accepted as efficacious

Table 1.2. Water medication in swine

Name of drug	Trade name (manufacturer)	Le-gend	With-drawal	Indications
Apramycin	Apralan (SmithKline Beecham)	OTC	28 days	Colibacillosis
Bacitracin	Solu-Tracin 200 (A.L. Labs)	OTC	0	Swine dysentery
Chlortetracycline	Aureomycin (Cyanamid)	OTC	1 day	Bacterial enteritis, bacterial pneumonia
Gentamicin	Garacin (Schering)	OTC	10 days	Colibacillosis, swine dysentery
Lincomycin	Lincomix (Upjohn)	OTC	6 days	Swine dysentery
Neomycin	Biosol, Neomix (Upjohn)	OTC	20 days	Bacterial diarrhea and enteritis
Sulfachlor-pyridazine	Vetisulid (Solvay)	OTC	4 days	Colibacillosis
Sulfamethazine	Sulmet (Cyanamid)	OTC	15 days	Bacterial pneumonia, colibacillosis
Tetracycline	Polyotic (Cyanamid)	OTC	7 days	Bacterial enteritis, bacterial pneumonia
Tiamulin	Denagard (Fermenta)	OTC	7 days	Swine dysentery, pleuropneumonia

Table 1.3. Injectable medication for swine

Name of drug	Trade name (manufacturer)	Legend	Withdrawal	Indications
Ceftiofur	Naxcel (Upjohn)	Rx	0	Bacterial pneumonia, salmonellosis
Erythromycin	Erythro-100 (200) (Sanofi)	OTC	7 days	Pneumonia, MMA, lepto, scours
Gentamicin	Garacin (Schering)	OTC	40 days	Colibacillosis
Lincomycin	Lincomix (Upjohn)	OTC	2 days	Mycoplasmal pneumonia, arthritis
Oxytetracycline	Liquamycin (Pfizer), others	OTC	28 days	Colibacillosis, pasteurellosis, lepto
Penicillin	several	OTC	7 days	Erysipelas
Tylosin	Tylan (Elanco)	OTC	14 days	Dysentery, pasteurella, arthritis, erysipelas

2

POLYSYSTEMIC DISEASES

ERYSIPELAS

ETIOLOGY:

A. Infectious—*Erysipelothrix rhusiopathiae* (formally *E. insidiosa*)
   1. Also causes disease in sheep and turkeys.
   2. Causes erysipeloid in humans.
B. Environmental and management factors
   1. Stress may precipitate disease (e.g., sudden changes in diet and/or temperature).
   2. Chronic low level aflatoxin exposure may increase susceptibility to disease.
C. Animal factors (immunity)
   1. Passive colostral immunity may last up to 3 months.
   2. Subclinical infection may induce active immunity.

EPIDEMIOLOGY:

A. 30-50% of healthy swine are carriers.
B. Organism is periodically shed in feces.
C. Contamination of water, food, and environment
D. Pigs are most susceptible to clinical disease between 3 months and 3 years of age.
E. Exposure to infected sheep and turkeys may increase risk of infection in swine.

PATHOGENESIS:

A. Entry via tonsilar or intestinal lymphoid tissue or via breaks in skin or mucous membrane
B. Septicemia

C. May localize to any body tissue, but especially to vascular endothelium (skin and heart) and joints.

CLINICAL SIGNS: May occur in any combination or not at all.

A. Acute
  1. Pyrexia—104°-108°F (40°-42°C)
  2. Depression
  3. Stilted gait
  4. Anorexia
  5. Diamond skin lesions—pathognomonic

B. Chronic
  1. Cardiac insufficiency—intolerance to exertion
  2. Lameness
  3. Enlarged joints

DIAGNOSIS:

A. Clinical signs—especially diamond skin lesions

B. Necropsy lesions
  1. Acute
    a. Widespread congestion, petechial and ecchymotic hemorrhages
    b. Microthrombi and focal necrosis
    c. Mononuclear inflammation
  2. Chronic
    a. Proliferative, nonsuppurative arthritis (hock, stifle, elbow, carpus)
    b. Serosanguineous synovial fluid
    c. Vegetative endocarditis

C. Culture
  1. Acute—blood, lungs, liver, spleen, lymph nodes, kidneys, joints
  2. Chronic—joints
  3. Take several samples from several pigs.

TREATMENT:

A. Antibiotics
  1. Penicillin—10,000 IU/lb. Drug of choice.
  2. Tetracyclines and tylosin are also effective.

B. Hyperimmune serum

C. Nothing works against chronic erysipelas.

PREVENTION AND CONTROL:

A. General sanitation

B. Immunization

1. Attenuated live—injectable or oral. Do not give with antiserum or antibiotics.
2. Bacterins—injectable
3. Give at weaning and every 6 months.
4. Vaccines do not prevent chronic erysipelas.

GLASSER'S DISEASE (HAEMOPHILUS POLYSEROSITIS)

ETIOLOGY: *Haemophilus parasuis*

EPIDEMIOLOGY:

A. Virulent and avirulent strains of the organism exist. Virulent strains usually belong to certain serological groups (Bakos group B; serotype 5). Infection with avirulent strains may protect against infection with virulent strains.
B. The organism is endemic in many herds—colonizes upper respiratory tract.
C. Disease is often very severe in specific pathogen free (SPF) or minimal disease pigs introduced into conventional herds.

PATHOGENESIS: Unknown, but probably:

A. Stress (weaning, transport, change in diet, change in temperature, etc.) compromises the immunologic status of the animal.
B. Endemic organisms become septicemic.
C. Organisms settle on serous and synovial membranes.

CLINICAL SIGNS:

A. Sudden onset; usually at 3-10 weeks of age in endemic herds. Minimal disease/SPF pigs may be affected at any age.
B. Acute fulminating septicemia may result in sudden death with few lesions.
C. Subacute or chronic infections result in pyrexia (105°-107°F [40.5°-41.6°C]), anorexia, labored breathing, lameness, swollen joints, and CNS signs (tremors, rear limb ataxia).
D. Rarely, infection has been associated with an acute myositis of the masseter muscles.

DIAGNOSIS:

A. Clinical signs
B. Necropsy

1. Fibrinous/serofibrinous pleuritis, pericarditis, peritonitis, arthritis, and meningitis
   a. Any combination of the above lesions
   b. Meningitis is most consistent; 80% of cases.
2. Histopathology—fibrinopurulent inflammation (mainly neutrophils)

C. Culture
1. Organism requires nicotinamide adenine dinucleotide (NAD).
2. *H. parasuis* can be isolated in only 35-57% of cases.

TREATMENT:

A. Must be early to be effective.
B. Initial treatment must be parenteral.
C. Infection is responsive to many antibiotics, e.g., penicillin, ampicillin, tetracyclines, tylosin, sulfas, others.

PREVENTION AND CONTROL:

A. Reduce stress.
B. Vaccination with a bacterin at time of greatest risk; usually at or shortly after weaning and again 3-4 weeks later.

PORCINE REPRODUCTIVE AND RESPIRATORY SYNDROME (PRRS)

SYNONYMS: Swine infertility and respiratory syndrome (SIRS), porcine epidemic abortion and respiratory syndrome (PEARS), mystery pig disease, blue ear disease

ETIOLOGY:

A. Lelystad or PRRS virus. This is an RNA virus related to lactase dehydrogenase-elevating virus (LDV), equine arteritis virus (EAV), and simian hemorrhagic fever virus (SHFV). These viruses would belong to a newly proposed arterivirus group.
B. Exposure to the fumonisin mycotoxin may increase the risk for the disease.

EPIDEMIOLOGY:

A. The syndrome was first reported in 1987. Large numbers of cases were reported in the summers of 1988 and 1989, especially from Indiana, Minnesota, and Iowa. A similar syndrome appeared in Europe in 1991. As more herds have become infected with the virus, the severity of the syndrome seems to have decreased.

B. The most common means of transmission appears to be via direct contact with an infected pig. Airborne transmission up to 2 miles and transmission via artificial insemination may also be possible.

C. Clinical disease appears to be milder in minimal disease herds. Some infected herds have no history of clinical disease.

PATHOGENESIS:

A. Although pathogenic mechanisms are poorly understood, it is supposed that the virus initially replicates in alveolar macrophages. Destruction of alveolar macrophages mediates inflammatory changes in the lung. A viremic stage allows infection of various organs, including the reproductive tract. The virus can cross the placenta and kill or weaken the fetus by an unknown mechanism.

B. Host antibody may enhance viral infection and replication in alveolar macrophages. Virus-antibody immune complexes are attracted to Fc receptors on macrophages but are not neutralized.

CLINICAL SIGNS:

A. Transient, mild anorexia, lethargy, and fever (103°- 105°F [39.5°-40.5°C]) in grower-finisher pigs and/or breeding animals.

B. Cyanosis of the ears (blue ear disease), vulva, tail, abdomen, or snout is occasionally reported.

C. Increased incidence of premature farrowings with small, weak, or stillborn piglets; and an increased incidence of fetal mummies.

D. Sows may show delayed or abnormal estrus cycles.

E. Respiratory distress, i.e., "thumping" and open-mouth breathing in suckling and recently weaned piglets. The incidence of other respiratory infections, e.g., *Pasteurella*, *Streptococcus*, *Haemophilus parasuis*, and *Salmonella* increases in young pigs. Preweaning mortality increases.

F. In some herds, chronic infection of nursery and grow/finish pigs may result in decreased growth rate and feed efficiency as well as increased morbidity and mortality from secondary infections.

G. Herd gradually returns to (almost) normal in 2-4 months.

DIAGNOSIS:

A. Clinical signs

B. Detection of viral antigen may be accomplished by virus isolation, fluorescent antibody, or immunoperoxidase staining.

C. Detection of viral antibodies in serum can be accomplished by immunoperoxidase monolayer assay (IPMA), indirect fluorescent antibody test (IFA), serum neutralization (SN), and enzyme-linked immunosorbant assay

(ELISA). The IFA is the most commonly used test in the United States. Paired samples are necessary because of a high prevalence of asymptomatic pigs and herds that are seropositive.

D. Typical respiratory lesions include interlobular edema, interstitial pneumonia characterized by Type II pneumocyte proliferation, and necrotizing alveolitis.

TREATMENT: None specific. Supportive therapy and prophylactic antibiotics to reduce secondary infections in surviving pigs would seem prudent.

PREVENTION AND CONTROL:

A. Avoidance; do not allow exposure to pigs from herds that have experienced the syndrome.
B. Change feed if positive for mycotoxins.
C. A vaccine (RespPRRS—Boehringer Ingelheim/Nobl Laboratories) has recently been approved.

Suggested Reading:

Christianson WT, Joo HS. 1994. Porcine reproductive and respiratory syndrome: A review. *Swine Health and Production* 2(2):10-28.

PSEUDORABIES

SYNONYMS: Aujeszky's Disease, infectious bulbar paralysis, mad itch

HISTORY: First described by Aujeszky in 1902

ETIOLOGY: Herpesvirus

EPIDEMIOLOGY:

A. Occurs worldwide; especially prevalent in localized areas of the midwestern and southeastern United States.
B. The pig is the natural host. While many other species are affected, practically all are dead-end hosts.
C. The primary route of spread of pseudorabies virus (PRV) is from infected to susceptible pigs.
D. Wild animals (especially raccoons and rodents) may become infected and transmit PRV from farm to farm.
E. Dogs, cats, and domestic ruminants are quite susceptible to, and uniformly die

from, PRV infection. Humans seem to be quite resistant.

F. PRV infection may become latent in swine. Recrudescence and viral shedding may occur in latently infected swine with no external signs.

G. PRV isolates apparently vary in virulence. Occasionally herds are infected but show mild or no clinical signs.

PATHOGENESIS:

PRV normally enters via nasal (aerosol) or oral (ingestion) passages—infects and replicates in upper respiratory epithelium—(a) travels up axoplasm of olfactory neurons to infect the CNS (thymidine kinase [TK] gene is involved)—(b) extends down the respiratory tract to infect epithelium of bronchial tree and alveoli—either CNS or respiratory infection may become viremic—virus infects other body tissues (reproductive tract).

CLINICAL SIGNS: Vary according to the age of pig affected. Also may vary in severity from herd to herd.

A. Baby piglets—preweaning
   1. Acute deaths, high morbidity. Mortality is often 100%. May be no signs preceding death.
   2. Pyrexia, depression, tremors, incoordination, and convulsions may precede death.
   3. Other inconsistent clinical signs include vomition and diarrhea or constipation.

B. Weanling and growing pigs
   1. Pneumonia, acute dry nonproductive cough, usually high morbidity, "flu-like" syndrome
   2. Pyrexia (up to 107°F [41.6°C]) and anorexia
   3. Vomition and constipation may be observed.
   4. Tremors, incoordination, and convulsions
   5. Mortality varies from up to 60% in nursery pigs to 0-15% in finishers.

C. Adults
   1. Infection may be inapparent.
   2. Pyrexia, anorexia, and pneumonia are the most common signs.
   3. Occasional CNS signs
   4. If a pregnant female is infected:
      a. Early embryonic death and resorption (0-30 days gestation)
      b. Abortion (40-90 days)
      c. Weak, stillborn, or macerated fetuses (>90 days)

DIAGNOSIS: If you make a tentative or positive diagnosis of PRV, notify your state veterinarian.

A. Clinical signs

B. Necropsy
   1. Few gross lesions
   2. May see congestion of meninges and nasal mucosa, congestion and petechial hemorrhages of lymph nodes and kidneys, pulmonary edema, necrotic foci on liver, spleen, and tonsil.
   3. Principal histologic lesion is a diffuse nonsuppurative meningoencephalomyelitis.
C. Virus isolation
D. Fluorescent antibody
E. Serology
   1. Serum neutralization (SN)
      a. SN is the standard regulatory test for PRV.
      b. Care must be taken in the collection of blood for SN as toxic serum can be a problem. Clean, sterile blood tubes and good venapucture technique is important.
   2. ELISA and latex agglutination are often used as screening tests. These tests can be performed rapidly and are highly sensitive.

TREATMENT:

A. None specific
B. Antibiotics may reduce secondary pneumonic infections in older animals.

PREVENTION: Directed toward prevention of infection in noninfected herds and prevention of clinical signs in infected herds.

A. Of infection
   1. Ideally, maintain closed herd.
   2. Purchase only animals that have tested negative or animals from qualified PRV-free herds.
   3. Isolate purchased animals for at least 2 weeks (preferably 30 days) and retest before introduction into the herd.
   4. Restrict access of wildlife and pets to the herd.
   5. Workers and visitors should be scrupulously clean, especially if they have access to other swine.
   6. Prevention of infection may be impossible for herds in highly endemic areas.
B. Of clinical signs—e.g., vaccination
   1. Vaccination is generally effective at reducing clinical signs of PRV, even in the face of an outbreak.
   2. Vaccination may not prevent infection, shedding, or latent infection with virulent virus.
   3. Vaccine use is regulated by state officials. Some states allow unrestricted use of vaccine, others allow vaccine use only in herds with a positive or tentative diagnosis of PRV or a high risk of exposure.

4. Types of vaccine
    a. Killed or inactivated
        i. Safe
        ii. Immunity may be weaker and shorter-lived than with MLV.
    b. Modified live or attenuated
        i. Good immunity
        ii. Vaccine virus may become latent.
        iii. Some concerns (minor) about reversion to virulence
        iv. May cause abortions or malformed fetuses if given to pregnant females.
    c. Genetically engineered vaccines. Several vaccines have been developed and approved that are based on a genetically altered viral strain. Typically one genetic alteration removes virulence; another provides for an antigenic marker to allow for a diagnostic test that can differentiate between vaccination titers and natural infection titers.

REGULATORY CONTROL: Varies some from state to state but generally:

A. All breeding swine over 6 months of age must test negative or be from a qualified negative herd prior to sale or show.
B. A qualified negative herd:
    1. Must initially test all animals over 6 months of age.
    2. To maintain qualified herd status, must test 25% of the herd every 3 months or 10% of the herd every month.
    3. All serological tests must be negative.
C. A percentage tested or monitored herd:
    1. Must test once a year.
    2. The percentage tested depends on herd size.
        a. In herds with 10 sows or fewer, all are tested.
        b. In herds with 11 to 35 sows, test 10.
        c. In herds with greater than 35 sows, test 30% up to a maximum of 30.
    3. Many states require monitored herd status to sell feeder pigs or cull sows and boars.
D. Positive swine may be sold only to slaughter or to quarantined feedlots.
E. Guidelines for individual herd eradication are available from the American Association of Swine Practitioners (AASP) and the Livestock Conservation Institute (LCI). Plans involve either total herd depopulation and repopulation, test and removal, or offspring segregation.

SALMONELLOSIS

ETIOLOGY: Three serotypes are generally associated with disease in swine.

A. *Salmonella choleraesuis* is by far the most common isolate from swine. It is associated with generalized septicemia, pneumonia, and enterocolitis.
B. *Salmonella typhimurium* is a less common isolate generally associated with enterocolitis.
C. *Salmonella typhisuis* is relatively rare cause of diarrhea, wasting, caseous lymphadenitis, and pneumonia.

EPIDEMIOLOGY:

A. *Salmonella* is present at a low-level endemic state in most herds. Asymptomatic carriers are common.
B. Clinical disease is often associated with some stress, e.g., ventilation problems, poor sanitation, overcrowding.
C. Disease occurs commonly in multiple-source feeder pigs.
D. *Salmonella* outbreaks are sometimes associated with immunosuppression, e.g., from eating aflatoxin-contaminated feed.
E. In many diagnostic laboratories, *Salmonella* is the second most common bacterial isolate from pneumonic swine lungs.
F. *Salmonella typhimurium* will infect and cause disease in humans. Although other serotypes could theoretically infect humans, they tend to be fairly well host-adapted to swine.

PATHOGENESIS:

A. The organism gains entry to the pig via fecal-oral contact.
B. The organism may invade the intestinal mucosa and become septicemic.
    1. Many of the clinical signs of septicemic salmonellosis are mediated by endotoxin.
    2. Septicemic infection often results in inflammation and necrosis of the lungs, liver, and spleen.
C. The organism may produce enterotoxins, which cause a hypersecretory diarrhea.
D. Endotoxins and other exotoxins are probably responsible for inflammation, vascular damage, and necrosis of the gut.

CLINICAL SIGNS:

A. Septicemic form
    1. Respiratory signs: dyspnea and cough
    2. Other signs of septicemia may be present; e.g., pyrexia, anorexia,

depression, purple discoloration of the skin, especially around the ears and ventral abdomen.

B. Gastrointestinal form
   1. Acute or chronic diarrhea, occasionally with blood
   2. Pyrexia, anorexia, and dehydration
   3. Signs may wax and wane within a herd.
   4. May occasionally see greatly distended abdomen due to rectal strictures.

DIAGNOSIS:

A. Clinical signs
B. Lesions—septicemic form
   1. Pneumonia with edema and hemorrhage. Fibrinous pleuritis also occurs commonly.
   2. Lesions suggestive of a septicemia are usually present, e.g., splenomegaly, hepatomegaly, hemorrhagic lymph nodes, ecchymotic renal hemorrhages, paratyphoid nodules in the liver.
   3. Enteric lesions are not consistently present.
C. Lesions—gastrointestinal form.
   1. Diffuse necrotic colitis and typhlitis. Usually some ileal involvement (compare to dysentery).
   2. Button ulcers
   3. Enlarged, hemorrhagic mesenteric lymph nodes
D. Culture
   1. *Salmonella choleraesuis* is readily cultured from the lungs, liver, and spleen of pigs with septicemia.
   2. Cultural enrichment (e.g., tetrathionate broth) is often necessary for fecal cultures.
   3. No culture technique will consistently identify subclinical carriers.

TREATMENT:

A. Antibiotics according to sensitivity
   1. Aminoglycosides—gentamicin (water), neomycin (feed and/or water)
      Recognize that aminoglycosides are poorly absorbed when given orally and are *extremely* persistent in tissues when given parenterally. Parenteral injection of gentamicin is approved only in neonatal pigs.
   2. Carbadox (feed)
   3. Ceftiofur (Naxcel) injection
   4. Injections of trimethoprim-sulfa (Tribrissen) are often effective against acute septicemic salmonellosis. This is an extra-label, non-approved drug use.
B. Feed and water antibiotics have limited efficacy when used on clinically ill animals. Their use should be viewed as prophylaxis rather than as treatment.

PREVENTION AND CONTROL:

A. Management (especially all-in, all-out pig flow) and sanitation
B. Vaccination
   1. Killed bacterins: Federally licensed *Salmonella* bacterins are available. These and autogenous bacterins may have limited efficacy in reducing clinical signs.
   2. Avirulent live vaccines: Injectable (Nitro-Sal, ARKO Laboratories) and intranasal (SC-54, Nobl Laboratories) avirulent *Salmonella choleraesuis* vaccines are available. These may stimulate a better cell-mediated immune response and offer greater protection than killed bacterins.
   3. A vaccine derived from an Re-17 mutagenically derived *Salmonella typhimurium* is approved for swine (ENDOVAC-Porci, IMMVAC, Inc.). This vaccine stimulates the production of anti-endotoxin antibodies. This may offer cross-protection against *Salmonella choleraesuis* and possibly other endotoxin-mediated diseases.

Suggested Reading:

Schwartz KJ. 1991. Diagnosing and controlling *Salmonella choleraesuis* in swine. *Vet Med* 86:1041-1048.

3

RESPIRATORY DISEASES

ATROPHIC RHINITIS (AR)

DEFINITION: Atrophic rhinitis is generally defined as a chronic, progressive disease of swine characterized by atrophy of the nasal turbinates (conchae). However, since the lesion of turbinate atrophy is not always associated with chronic, progressive disease, some have recommended that the term *progressive atrophic rhinitis* be used to describe the disease.

ETIOLOGY: AR is a *multifactorial* disease. Virtually any agent that can irritate the nasal mucosa can produce an inflammatory response that will disturb the growth of the nasal turbinates.

A. Infectious factors
  1. *Bordetella bronchiseptica* (Bb)
     a. Consistently causes turbinate atrophy in experimental infections.
     b. Pure Bb infections (uncomplicated by secondary invaders) are self-limiting. Lesions heal; there is little or no effect on performance.
     c. There are strain differences in AR pathogenicity related to adhesion and toxin production.
  2. *Pasteurella multocida* (Pm)
     a. Some strains of Pm (usually capsular type D, more rarely type A) produce a thermolabile, dermonecrotic toxin. This toxin induces severe, persistent turbinate atrophy; it may also cause liver and kidney damage. This toxin may be the most important virulence factor for the production of severe, progressive AR.
     d. Bb and Pm together consistently produce a more severe, more persistent turbinate atrophy than either agent alone.
  3. *Haemophilus parasuis*
     a. May cause mild turbinate atrophy.

b. May potentiate the pathogenic effects of Pm and/or Bb.

4. Cytomegalovirus (Inclusion Body Rhinitis—IBR)
   a. Does *not* cause turbinate atrophy.
   b. May damage the nasal mucosa, thereby enhancing colonization by other bacterial pathogens.

B. Environmental factors
1. Ammonia at 50-100 ppm will exacerbate lesions associated with Bb infection.
2. Any environmental or social stressor will exacerbate AR, i.e., crowding, chilling, inadequate ventilation, drafts, dust, etc.
3. Nutrition. At one time, AR was thought to be caused by an imbalance of calcium and phosphorus in the diet. Although this theory has been largely discredited, suboptimal nutrition should be considered as another stressor that can exacerbate AR.

C. Animal factors
1. Age of dam: Litters farrowed by older sows are generally less severely affected than are gilt litters. Older sows have had more exposure to pathogenic organisms and can pass a higher level of passive immunity on to their baby pigs.
2. Genetic factors: Certain breeds (Hampshires and Durocs) may be more susceptible. Heritability of turbinate atrophy has been estimated at 15%.
3. Concurrent diseases: Scours, pneumonia, mange, etc. Some have theorized that turbinate atrophy is more a symptom than a cause of poor health and performance.

EPIDEMIOLOGY:

A. Transmission
1. The piglet probably acquires the infectious agents from nose to nose contact with a chronically infected dam.
2. Horizontal transmission of infectious agents among young pigs also occurs.
3. Cats and rats may carry the infectious agents. This is probably of minor significance compared to pig-to-pig transmission.
4. In general, the younger a pig is infected, the more likely it is to develop AR.

B. Prevalence
1. From 50% to 75% of market hogs have at least mild lesions of turbinate atrophy.
2. Nationwide, probably 80% of swine herds are affected to some degree by turbinate atrophy.
3. Incidence and severity of turbinate atrophy peaks in hogs slaughtered during the spring and summer months. Presumably, this is because these pigs were exposed to a harsh wintertime environment (minimal ventilation) when they were most susceptible (neonates and weanlings).

CLINICAL SIGNS:

A. Mild lesions of turbinate atrophy (observed at necropsy or slaughter check) are common and are seldom associated with clinical signs. Mild lesions have little or no effect on the overall health and performance of pigs.

B. The presence of clinical signs (especially later ones) usually indicate severe disease. Severe lesions are often associated with poor growth performance.

1. Early clinical signs (nursery; young growers)
   a. Sneezing, sniffling
   b. Mucopurulent nasal exudate
2. Later clinical signs (growers and finishers)
   a. Twisted or shortened snouts
   b. Excessive lacrimation with tear stains at the medial canthus (due to blockage of the nasolacrimal duct)
   c. Epistaxis
   d. Decreased growth rate—up to 20%
   e. Increased feed/gain ratio

PATHOGENESIS:

The piglet is inoculated with Bb soon after birth from a carrier dam—Bb attaches to and colonizes the nasal epithelium—Bb toxins diffuse through the submucosa and induce local inflammation and degenerative changes in osteoblasts—damaged mucosa allows Pm to colonize and produce toxins—the combined effect of toxins on osteogenic cells produces turbinate atrophy and disturbed growth of the maxilla—Pm toxins may also damage the liver and other internal organs.

As mentioned earlier, any irritant may induce mild changes in the nasal turbinates. Mild changes, however, are usually of little or no consequence to the overall health and performance of the pig. Toxigenic Pm and/or Bb are often present in herds with severe, growth-retarding AR. However, toxigenic Pm has been isolated from herds with no clinical signs of AR and only mild lesions of turbinate atrophy. Management of environment, nutrition, and concurrent disease is usually optimal in these herds.

DIAGNOSIS:

A. Clinical signs

B. Nasal culture

1. The presence of Bb and/or Pm in nasal swabs supports a diagnosis of AR but is not by itself definitively diagnostic of the disease.
2. One is more likely to detect these bacteria if the ethmoidal area is cultured (i.e., the further back, the better). Pm is found in the tonsil frequently when it cannot be found in the nose.
3. Selective media are described for the isolation of Bb and Pm (*J Clin Microbiol* 1993, 31:364-367).

4. Pm toxin may be identified by its ability to produce dermonecrosis in guinea pigs, lethality in mice, and cytotoxicity in embryonic bovine lung cell culture.

C. Necropsy and slaughter checks.
 1. Allow for definitive assessment of turbinate atrophy.
 2. One should examine at least 20 pigs to get an accurate impression of the prevalence of turbinate atrophy within a herd.
 3. Saw the snout in cross-section at the level of the second premolar (the first cheek tooth if <5 months; the second cheek tooth if >5 months).
 4. Grade the severity of the lesions.
  a. Some controversy exists as to the "best" grading system.
  b. The grading system in most common use is based on the amount of space between the ventral turbinate and the floor of the nasal cavity (Table 3.1).
  c. With any grading system, the most useful herd parameter is the percentage of animals with moderate and severe lesions (≥AR score 3 if you are using Table 3.1).
  d. A grading system is useful for comparing herds and assessing response to therapy. Keep in mind that AR lesion scores will vary with the seasons (highest in the spring and summer).

Table 3.1 Scale for scoring turbinate atrophy

Total turbinate space left and right (mm)	Score	Interpretation
0 to 2	1[a]	Negative
3 to 6	0	Negative
7 to 9	1	Negative
10 to 12	2	Suspect
13 to 16	3	Positive
17 to 20	4	Positive
≥ 21	5	Positive

Source: From Straw BE, et al., *J Am Vet Med Assoc* 1983, 182:607-11.

Note: 1/2 point is added to the score for turbinate asymmetry and for septal deviation. Maximum total score = 5.

[a] 3 to 6 mm of space is considered to exist in the normal pig. When there is less than 3 mm of space, inflammation or collapse of the turbinates may have occurred.

TREATMENT AND CONTROL:

The objective of treatment and control measures in most commercial herds is the reduction of economic losses due to the disease. Losses may be minimal with mild turbinate atrophy. However, the objective for seedstock herds may be total freedom from lesions of turbinate atrophy and absence of infection with Bb and toxigenic Pm.

A. Chemotherapeutics
   1. Several feed medications containing tetracyclines and/or sulfonamides are labeled for "maintaining rate of gain in the presence of atrophic rhinitis." Other feed medications may also help reduce the adverse effects of AR. Antibiotics given through feed or water have little direct effect on the infectious agents of AR. The beneficial effects of antibiotics are likely due to growth promotion and improved overall health.
   2. Several programs of intensive parenteral medication of neonates have evolved in an attempt to eliminate the causative organisms; e.g., 200 mg LA-200 (oxytetracycline) at 1, 7, 14, and 21 days; Naxcel (ceftiofur) at 10 mg at day 1, 20 mg at day 7, 40 mg at weaning; others.

B. Vaccination
   1. Bb and Pm bacterins/toxoids
      a. Most products are recommended to be given twice to the sow prefarrowing; some also recommend piglet vaccination.
      b. Sow vaccination (colostral immunity) is probably more important than piglet vaccination.
      c. Pm toxoid is both immunogenic and protective. As this is an important virulence factor, vaccines should definitely contain this component.
   2. Modified live intranasal Bb vaccine to piglets. These avirulent Bb are reported to compete with virulent Bb for binding sites and thus prevent the initial insult which leads to AR.

C. Management
   1. All-in, all-out farrowing and nursery with thorough sanitation between groups.
   2. Reduce stress and crowding, especially in nursery.
   3. Provide an optimal air environment. This may include improved ventilation, decreased levels of ammonia and dust in the air, and improved temperature control. Consultation with other experts may be necessary.
   4. Control concurrent disease, especially parasitism, scours, pneumonia.
   5. Farrow older sows, for less vertical transmission of infectious agents, increased immunity.
   6. Provide adequate nutrition, especially easily digestible starter/nursery diets.
   7. Do not allow cats and rats in swine buildings.

D. Eradication
   1. The most effective way to eradicate AR from a herd is complete depopula-

tion and repopulation with AR-free swine. This is probably not necessary in many herds with mild turbinate atrophy. It should be considered if there are concurrent diseases (e.g., pseudorabies, dysentery, mycoplasma pneumonia) that are difficult to control and if the genetic base of the herd needs upgrading anyway.

2. AR may be eradicated from herds which need to preserve their genetic base (i.e., seedstock herds) via the SPF program (caesarian delivery, raised in isolation) or segregated early weaning (SEW).

E. Disease monitoring. Whatever control measures are implemented, the disease must be monitored to assess efficacy and cost benefit. Useful parameters include days to market, percentage light-weight market hogs; feed:gain ratio, AR lesion score (Table 3.1).

INCLUSION BODY RHINITIS

ETIOLOGY: Cytomegalovirus (herpes)

EPIDEMIOLOGY:

A. Infection is widespread; subclinical disease is common.
B. Virus is spread primarily via respiratory secretions.
C. Expression of clinical disease depends on the immune status of the dam and the age of her pigs at infection.
D. Clinical disease occurs almost exclusively in pigs less than 4 weeks old.

CLINICAL SIGNS:

A. Sneezing, snorting
B. Purulent or serous nasal discharge
C. Open mouth breathing; obstruction of the airway with exudate
D. Occasional deaths due to suffocation
E. Infection of the pregnant sow may result in an increase in stillborn and weak pigs.

DIAGNOSIS:

A. Clinical signs
B. Gross pathology
   1. Petechia and edema of the lungs and subcutaneous tissues
   2. Abundant mucopurulent nasal exudate from secondary infections is common.
C. Histopathology: large basophilic intranuclear inclusions in nasal epithelium

D. Virus isolation and serological tests (indirect immunofluorescence, ELISA)

TREATMENT: None effective. May give antibiotics for secondary bacterial infection.

PREVENTION AND CONTROL: None. Outbreaks are usually self-limiting.

NECROTIC RHINITIS

SYNONYMS: Proliferative rhinitis, bullnose

ETIOLOGY: *Fusobacterium necrophorum*

EPIDEMIOLOGY:

A. Most commonly seen in young pigs.
B. Associated with poor sanitation, especially in cutting needle teeth.

CLINICAL SIGNS:

A. Slowly progressive swelling and abscessation of snout
B. Depression, anorexia, and dyspnea

DIAGNOSIS: Usually obvious—gross evidence of abscessation

TREATMENT: Probably useless, but surgical debridement and antibiotics could be used.

PREVENTION AND CONTROL: Good sanitation

SWINE INFLUENZA

HISTORY: First observed in 1918, coincident with a human influenza pandemic.

ETIOLOGY: Type A influenza virus

EPIDEMIOLOGY:

A. Influenza viruses are classified by hemagglutinin (H) and neuraminidase (N) surface antigens. Most U.S. strains are of the H1N1 subtype; H3N2 subtypes are common in other parts of the world.
B. Usually introduced to a farm via movement of animals (purchase of breeding stock, feeder pigs, show animals).
C. Transmitted from pig to pig by nasopharyngeal route.
D. Virus may be maintained in asymptomatic carrier pigs.
E. Virus may be transmitted between pigs and humans. Though uncommon, at least 2 human deaths have been attributed to exposure to influenza-infected swine since 1988.

PATHOGENESIS:

A. Virus attaches to respiratory epithelial cells via the hemagglutinin protein on envelope of virus.
B. Enters cells and replicates rapidly.
C. Causes degenerative changes, necrosis, and inflammation throughout the respiratory tract.

CLINICAL SIGNS:

A. Most clinical outbreaks occur in late autumn and early winter. Outbreaks may be precipitated by wide fluctuations in temperature (greater than 15°-20°F [8°-11°C] over 24 hours).
B. Sudden onset, up to 100% morbidity
C. Paroxysmal coughing. Cough is deep, dry, and nonproductive.
D. Anorexia.
E. Pyrexia, up to 108°F (42°C)
F. Rapid and complete recovery in 10 to 14 days, practically no mortality if uncomplicated by secondary or concurrent disease.
G. Signs may be exacerbated by concurrent disease (ascariasis, mycoplasmal pneumonia, pasteurellosis, *Actinobacillus* pleuropneumonia, etc.).
H. Sows and gilts infected during pregnancy may farrow small, poorly viable litters.

DIAGNOSIS:

A. Clinical signs
B. Lesions are rarely observed; few pigs die of uncomplicated swine influenza.
    1. Gross lesions: hyperemia of lungs and airway, anterioventral lobular consolidation
    2. Microscopic lesions: congestion; lobular atelectasis, emphysema in other lobules; mixed inflammatory reaction
C. Virus isolation

D. Fluorescent antibody
E. Paired serology
   1. The protective antigen is the hemagglutinin protein.
   2. Serologic test is hemagglutination inhibition.
   3. Must demonstrate a rise in titer for diagnosis, as many normal swine will have antibody.
   4. Maternal antibody may persist for 2-4 months.
F. Exclusion of other diagnoses (especially pseudorabies)

TREATMENT:

A. None specific
B. Nursing care
   1. Comfortable environment
   2. Minimal stresses
C. Antibacterial drugs in drinking water to prevent or control secondary bacterial infections.

PREVENTION AND CONTROL:

A. Control synergistic diseases: mycoplasma, pasteurella, ascariasis, etc.
B. An influenza vaccine has recently been approved for swine (MaxiVac-Flu, Syntrovet).
C. Minimize exposure by maintaining a closed herd.
D. Veterinarians have a responsibility to protect human health. Swine showing clinical signs of influenza should *not* be allowed at public exhibitions or sales.

PULMONARY BORDETELLOSIS

SYNONYM: Whooping cough

ETIOLOGY: *Bordetella bronchiseptica*

EPIDEMIOLOGY:

A. The organism is probably carried in the nasal cavity of an asymptomatic carrier sow.
B. Horizontal transmission among piglets may occur.
C. Clinical disease occurs only in very young pigs.

PATHOGENESIS:

A. The organism colonizes bronchi and bronchioles.
B. Bacterial products (probably both endotoxins and exotoxins) diffuse into the lung tissue causing vascular damage and fibrosis.

CLINICAL SIGNS:

A. Coughing in nursing or recently weaned piglets
B. Mild fever, up to 104°F (40°C)
C. Anorexia
D. Mortality up to 30%
E. May or may not be signs of rhinitis

DIAGNOSIS:

A. Clinical signs
B. Lesions
   1. Gross: anterioventral hemorrhagic consolidation in a lobular (checker-board) pattern; may have fibrinous pleuritis.
   2. Microscopic
      a. Acute: hemorrhage, edema, vasculitis
      b. Chronic: endothelial hypertrophy and hyperplasia, adventitial hyperplasia, pulmonary fibrosis
C. Bacterial culture

TREATMENT:

A. Antibiotics according to sensitivity: oxytetracycline, sulfonamides, others

PREVENTION AND CONTROL: Vaccination with *Bordetella* bacterins

MYCOPLASMAL POLYSEROSITIS

ETIOLOGY: *Mycoplasma hyorhinis*

EPIDEMIOLOGY:

A. Probably spread via aerosol and contact.
B. Intranasal and pneumonic infection is common, even without clinical disease. "Outbreaks" of clinical disease are relatively uncommon.

PATHOGENESIS:

A. Organism colonizes upper respiratory tract.
B. Stress precipitates a septicemia.
C. Organism settles on serous and synovial membranes.

CLINICAL SIGNS:

A. Usually occur between 3-10 weeks of age.
B. Moderate fever, 104°-105°F (40°-40.6°C)
C. Anorexia
D. Arched back, tucked-up abdomen
E. Labored breathing
F. Lameness, swollen joints
   Acute signs abate after 2 weeks, but lameness may persist for 2-3 months.
G. Morbidity, up to 25%; mortality, low

DIAGNOSIS:

A. Clinical signs
B. Necropsy
   1. Serofibrinous/seropurulent polyserositis—i.e., pleuritis, pericarditis, peritonitis—and arthritis (any or all of the above lesions)
   2. Histopathology: lymphocytic infiltration
C. Joint culture

TREATMENT: Although the organism is sensitive to tylosin and lincomycin, nothing works clinically.

PREVENTION AND CONTROL: Avoid precipitating stresses.

A. Concurrent respiratory or enteric disease
B. Extreme temperature variation
C. Moving, crowding, etc.

PLEUROPNEUMONIA

ETIOLOGY: *Actinobacillus pleuropneumoniae* (sometimes abbreviated APP), previously known as *Haemophilus pleuropneumoniae*

EPIDEMIOLOGY:

A. Clinical disease seems to be associated with intensive swine production.
B. Recovered swine can be chronic carriers. This is often the means of introduction of the disease into a herd.
C. Serotypes 1, 3, 4, 5, 7, 8, and 9 have been identified in the United States; serotypes 1, 5, and 7 are the most common isolates.
D. In an Iowa survey, 32% of breeding stock and 68.8% of swine herds had serologic evidence of infection. Surveys in other parts of the United States and Canada have shown similar or higher prevalence rates.

PATHOGENESIS:

A. Stress (crowding, transport, chilling) may trigger clinical disease.
B. Strains vary in virulence. Virulence factors include:
   1. Capsule: may help the bacteria evade body defenses, e.g., opsonization and phagocytosis. Strains with thicker capsules may be more virulent.
   2. Lipopolysaccharide (endotoxin): has many biological effects, one of which is to stimulate the release of inflammatory mediators. Pigs can die acutely of endotoxic shock.
   3. Exotoxins: especially hemolysins and cytolysins. These may lyse phagocytic cells and thus mediate tissue damage and necrosis.

CLINICAL SIGNS:

A. Peracute form: sudden death with no other clinical signs.
B. Acute form: characterized by anorexia, depression, pyrexia (up to 107°F, 41.7°C). May or may not see labored breathing and coughing. Death may occur within 24-36 hours after onset of clinical signs.
C. Chronic form: characterized by intermittent cough, poor appetite and decreased weight gains. For every 1% of hogs in a finishing group with gross evidence of pleuritis at slaughter, the whole group is estimated to take 1.2 days longer to reach market weight.

DIAGNOSIS:

A. Clinical signs
B. Lesions
   1. Acute
      a. Pulmonary hemorrhage, edema, and/or necrosis (firm and friable)
      b. Lesions are distributed throughout the lung; possibly more severe in the caudal (diaphragmatic) lung lobes.
      c. Fibrinous pleuritis and/or pleural effusion
   2. Chronic
      a. Encapsulated, abscesslike nodules

b. Fibrinous or fibrous pleuritis with pleural adhesions

C. Culture
1. Organism requires nicotinamide adenine dinucleotide (NAD) for growth.
   a. Cross-streaking a blood agar isolation plate with a nonhemolytic *Staphylococcus epidermidis* (which produces NAD) will allow the growth of the organism near the *Staph* streak (satellite phenomenon).
   b. Media supplemented with NAD (chocolate agar) may be used.
2. Small, beta-hemolytic colonies
3. Rapid inoculation of suitable culture media is important since the organism often dies in transport media.
4. In mixed infections, APP is often overgrown by other organisms, especially *P. multocida*.

D. Serology
1. Several serologic tests have been described; however, complement fixation (CF) is the most commonly available. The CF test has a high specificity and low sensitivity, which limits its usefulness in identifying individual infected animals. It is useful in identifying infection within a group when a number of animals can be tested.
2. Antibodies decline rapidly, therefore positive titers suggest recent infection.

TREATMENT:

A. Acute
1. Parenteral antibiotics
   a. Ceftiofur (Naxcel—Upjohn): 3-5 mg/kg once daily for 3 days
   b. Procaine penicillin G: up to 10 times the label dose of 3,000 IU/lb may be necessary.
   c. Extra-label drugs that may be effective: ampicillin, spectinomycin, trimethoprim-sulfa, sulfachlorpyridazine.
   d. Many strains are resistant to tetracyclines.
2. Tiamulin (Denagard—Fermenta) at 180 ppm in drinking water

B. Chronic: Nothing works.

PREVENTION AND CONTROL:

A. Vaccination
1. Commercially available vaccines are whole cell bacterins.
2. Pigs should be vaccinated once at 5-6 weeks of age and again 2-4 weeks later.
3. Most commercial bacterins contain serotypes 1, 5, and 7.
4. Bacterins are effective at reducing death losses due to pleuropneumonia; they are not as effective at preventing chronic disease.
5. Some products have been associated with abscesses at the injection site.

6. Paraffin oil adjuvanted vaccines may be more effective at reducing lesions and improving gain in chronic herds than are aluminum hydroxide adjuvanted vaccines.
7. Autogenous bacterins may be effective in certain herds when commercial vaccines are not effective.

B. As the disease seems to be associated with environmental and other stresses, minimizing these will help.
C. If a herd is seronegative, replacement stock should be obtained from another seronegative herd.
D. The disease can potentially be eliminated from a herd by segregated early weaning.

Suggested reading:

Fedorka-Cray PJ, Hoffman L, Cray WC, Gray JT, Breisch SA, and Anderson GA. 1993. *Actinobacillus (Haemophilus) pleuropneumoniae*. Part I. History, epidemiology, serotyping, and treatment. *Compend Contin Educ Pract Vet* 15:1447-1455.

Fedorka-Cray PJ, Anderson GA, Cray WC, Gray JT, and Breisch SA. 1994. *Actinobacillus (Haemophilus) pleuropneumoniae*. Part II. Virulence factors, immunity, and vaccines. *Compend Contin Educ Pract Vet* 16:117-125.

Tubbs RC. 1988. Managing the swine herd that's been infected with *Haemophilus pleuropneumoniae*. *Vet Med* 83:220-229.

MYCOPLASMAL PNEUMONIA

SYNONYMS: Enzootic pneumonia, virus pig pneumonia

ETIOLOGY: *Mycoplasma hyopneumoniae*

EPIDEMIOLOGY:

A. *Mycoplasma hyopneumoniae* is the most common cause of chronic pneumonia in swine.
B. In a Missouri survey, 68% of hogs slaughtered in the winter and 56% of hogs slaughtered in the summer had lesions typical of mycoplasmal pneumonia.
C. Most herds are affected to some degree.
D. Organisms are carried by chronically infected swine.

PATHOGENESIS:

A. The organism is spread via contact and aerosols.

B. The organism colonizes the cilia of the trachea, bronchi, and bronchioles.
C. Mucociliary clearance is reduced.
D. The organism causes peribronchial lymphoreticular hyperplasia.
E. Mild, uncomplicated cases of mycoplasmal pneumonia will spontaneously resolve. However, other bacterial infections (*Pasteurella multocida*, *Streptococcus suis*, *Actinobacillus pleuropneumoniae*, *Salmonella choleraesuis*) often occur due to compromised pulmonary defenses.
F. Economically significant disease is often associated with poor environment, continuous flow production, overcrowding, and other stressors.

CLINICAL SIGNS:

A. Usually not evident until pigs are 3-6 months old.
B. Chronic, nonproductive cough; usually induced by exercise.
C. Decreased growth rate; for every 10% of lung affected by pneumonia, average daily gain is reduced by 5.3%.
D. Anorexia and pyrexia are not noted in uncomplicated disease.
E. Morbidity is variable and mortality is low in uncomplicated disease.
F. Secondary bacterial infections commonly exacerbate clinical signs.

DIAGNOSIS:

A. Clinical signs
B. Gross lesions
    1. Purple to gray consolidation
    2. Anterioventral distribution
    3. Lobar pattern
C. Microscopic lesions
    1. Perivascular and peribronchial lymphocytic infiltration
    2. Lymphoid hyperplasia
    3. Mainly mononuclear inflammation
D. Culture of the organism is possible but difficult.
E. Fluorescent antibody tests on lung tissue
F. Serologic tests have been described but are not commonly used.

TREATMENT:

A. Several feed and water antimicrobials have been shown to reduce the severity of pneumonia and improve performance.
    1. Lincomycin (Lincomix) at 200 g/ton of feed for 21 days. This is the only label approved feed additive for mycoplasmal pneumonia.
    2. Tetracyclines
    3. Tylosin (Tylan)
    4. Tiamulin (Denagard)
B. Improving management and environment may significantly influence a

pneumonia problem.

1. All-in, all-out rearing throughout the grow/finish period is probably the most important management technique for control of pneumonia.
2. Draft-free environment, comfortable temperature
3. Freedom from noxious gases, especially ammonia

PREVENTION AND CONTROL:

A. Improved management and environment
B. Minimal disease systems, e.g., SPF, SEW
C. Several vaccines are available. Vaccination may reduce lesions and improve gains.

PASTEURELLOSIS

ETIOLOGY: *Pasteurella multocida*

EPIDEMIOLOGY:

A. *Pasteurella multocida* is the most common bacterial isolate from pneumonic swine lungs. Capsular type A strains are most common.
B. The organism is a common inhabitant of the upper respiratory tract of swine.
C. The organism can be transmitted by contact or aerosols.

PATHOGENESIS:

A. *Pasteurella multocida* is an opportunistic pathogen.
   1. The normal healthy swine lung is quite resistant to infection with *P. multocida.*
   2. Other infections that impair pulmonary defense mechanisms (mycoplasma, ascarid migration, influenza, etc.) render the lung susceptible to infection with *P. multocida.*
B. The effects of *P. multocida* infection are due to extensive inflammatory reaction (decreasing functional lung tissue) and endotoxin absorption.

CLINICAL SIGNS: Vary according to the severity of infection.

A. Dyspnea ("thumping" respiratory movement)
B. Moist, productive cough
C. Anorexia
D. Pyrexia, up to 107°F (41.7°C)
E. Morbidity and mortality is variable. Some pigs die of acute disease; some that

recover become poor doers.

DIAGNOSIS:

A. Clinical signs
B. Lesions
   1. Purulent bronchopneumonia—gross lesions are the same as for mycoplasma pneumonia (anterioventral distribution, lobar pattern); in addition, creamy pus is often present in the bronchi and bronchioles.
   2. Severe cases may have fibrinous pleuritis and pericarditis.
C. Culture

TREATMENT: Antibiotics based on sensitivity

A. Clinically ill animals should be treated parenterally. Possible choices include ampicillin, ceftiofur, erythromycin, oxytetracycline, penicillin, and tylosin.
B. *Pasteurella multocida* is resistant to streptomycin, sulfonamides, and lincomycin.

PREVENTION AND CONTROL:

A. As pasteurellosis is almost always a secondary infection, identification and control of the primary problem (mycoplasma, parasites, etc.) is necessary.
B. Vaccination with *P. multocida* bacterins may have some protective effect.
C. Feed or water medications (tetracyclines, tylosin, sulfonamides) may have a protective effect.
D. Improved environmental management
E. All-in, all-out rearing

VERMINOUS PNEUMONIA

ETIOLOGY: *Ascaris suum*
Metastrongylus elongatus (lungworm)

EPIDEMIOLOGY:

A. More common in pasture-raised swine; however, ascarids can also be a problem in confinement.
B. Ascarids have a direct life cycle; the lungworm requires an earthworm as an intermediate host.

PATHOGENESIS:

A. Ascarids
   1. After larvated eggs hatch in the small intestine, larvae migrate through the liver and lungs.
   2. In the lungs, larvae break through capillaries into alveoli and migrate up the airways.
   3. Lung migration induces alveolar collapse, hemorrhage, and local inflammation.
   4. Ascarids tend to have a more severe impact on pig performance the earlier the pig is infected.

B. Lungworms
   1. Swine ingest infective larvae in an earthworm.
   2. Larvae migrate to mesenteric lymph nodes, right heart, and lungs.
   3. Adults mature in the bronchioles of the diaphragmatic lung lobes.

CLINICAL SIGNS:

A. Dyspnea
B. "Thumping," especially with ascarids
C. Unthriftiness

DIAGNOSIS:

A. Clinical signs
B. Lesions
   1. Ascarids
      a. White spots on liver
         i. Focal reaction to migrating larvae
         ii. The number and severity of liver spots is not correlated with the severity of ascarid infection.
         iii. White spots regress 35 to 42 days postinfection.
      b. Adult worms in intestine
   2. Lungworms—adults in bronchioles
   3. Both ascarids and lungworms—emphysema and edema, especially in diaphragmatic lobes
C. Fecal flotation: Verminous pneumonia may be present with no parasite eggs evident in feces.

TREATMENT AND CONTROL:

A. Sanitation
   1. The McLean County Sanitation System, developed in 1927 yet still sound advice.
      a. Farrowing pens or houses should be cleaned and disinfected before

farrowing time.

b. The sow should be scrubbed with soap and water thoroughly before being placed in the dry pen or house.

c. The sow and pigs should be hauled to a "clean" pen or pasture at the appropriate time.

d. Old hog lots or permanent pastures should not be used.

B. Anthelmintics

1. Ascarids

a. Ascarids are sensitive to a wide variety of anthelmintics (piperazine, hygromycin B, dichlorvos, levamisole, pyrantel, ivermectin, fenbendazole).

b. Therapy must be directed toward the whole herd (reduce shedding of ova), since larval stages are responsible for damage.

c. Continuous feeding of pyrantel tartrate (Banminth) will block larval migration.

2. Lungworms are sensitive to levamisole, fenbendazole, and ivermectin.

3. If parasites are present on the farm:

a. Sows should be dewormed 5 to 10 days before breeding and again 5 to 10 days before farrowing.

b. Boars should be dewormed twice at 30 day intervals upon arrival at the farm and every 6 months thereafter.

c. Pigs should be dewormed at 5 to 6 weeks of age and again 30 days later if not on continuous pyrantel feeding.

4

GASTROINTESTINAL DISEASES

COLIBACILLOSIS

ETIOLOGY: enterotoxigenic *Escherichia coli* (ETEC)

EPIDEMIOLOGY:

A. Non-enterotoxigenic *E. coli* are normal gut inhabitants.
B. ETEC is the most important primary cause of diarrhea in piglets less than 5 days of age.
C. Pathogenic strains are usually characterized by certain fimbrial adhesins (F4 [K88], F5 [K99], F6 [987P], and F41) and the production of enterotoxins (STa, STb, LT).
D. *E. coli* may contribute to diarrhea in older nursing piglets or weaned pigs.
    1. Pure infections are rare. Viral and coccidial infections are usually also present.
    2. Antigenic association of strains with disease is not as clear-cut as in neonatal disease.
E. Invasive strains may cause septicemia.
F. A sow probably harbors and periodically sheds pathogenic strains; however, the main route of spread is through fecal contamination by other scouring piglets.
G. Poor sanitation and/or continuous-flow farrowing rooms contribute to the build up of ETEC in the environment.

PATHOGENESIS:

E. coli enters piglet orally and adheres to receptors on epithelial cells of small intestine via fimbria. The bacterium produces heat-labile (LT) and/or heat-stable (ST) enterotoxins. LT stimulates the enzyme adenyl cyclase, which causes an increase in intracellular cyclic AMP. This stimulates an increased secretion of bicarbonate, sodium, and water into gut lumen, which results in diarrhea, dehydration, acidosis, and hyperkalemia. The dehydration and electrolyte disturbances are often the cause of death. ST produces a similar hypersecretory diarrhea via the stimulation of guanylate cyclase, which causes an increase in intracellular cyclic GMP.

CLINICAL SIGNS:

A. Clear watery to yellowish-brown pasty diarrhea
B. Dehydration
C. Depression, gauntness, inflamed perineum
D. Variable death loss; higher in younger piglets

DIAGNOSIS:

A. Clinical signs
B. pH of feces: alkaline ($\geq$8)
C. Culture of small intestine
    1. Number of organisms
    2. Smooth colony types on Tergitol 7
    3. Isolates can be characterized by fimbrial antigens and enterotoxin production.
    4. Ligated loop test for enteropathogenicity
D. Histopathology: lack of villus atrophy
E. Gross pathology: distended gas-filled intestine, villi intact, chyle in mesenteric lymphatics

TREATMENT:

A. Antibacterial drugs, e.g., gentamicin, neomycin, sulfachlorpyridizine, spectinomycin, apramycin, ampicillin, oxytetracycline, trimethoprim-sulfa (not approved), others
B. Oral *E. coli* antiserum
C. Fluid and electrolyte therapy
    1. Oral: Resorb—SmithKline Beecham; Bluelite—TechMix, Inc.; others
    2. Parenteral: usually NaCl and $NaHCO_3$ i.p.
    3. Water acidifiers

PREVENTION AND CONTROL:

A. Management
    1. Warm and dry environment
    2. All-in, all-out farrowing rooms
    3. Sanitation: power washing, easily cleanable surfaces
B. Vaccination of sow
    1. Kohler milk vaccine.
        a. A live culture of a farm- specific strain of ETEC grown in milk and

top-dressed on the gestating sow's feed.

b. This stimulates a good secretory antibody (IgA) response in the sow; therefore, antibodies should be present in both colostrum and milk.

c. This also has the danger of exposing the baby piglets to live, virulent ETEC. Sows should be dosed at least 3 weeks prior to farrowing to allow time for fecal shedding to decrease. Sows should be dosed in a separate facility from the farrowing area and washed before being moved to the farrowing area.

2. Commercial bacterins and subunit pilus vaccines
   a. Parenterally administered vaccines tend to stimulate more of a humoral (IgG) antibody response; therefore, significant passive antibody transfer can occur only through the colostrum.
   b. Specific pilus antigens for most enteropathogenic strains are present in commercial vaccines.
   c. Commercial vaccines are usually efficacious against colibacillosis affecting piglets less than 5 days of age.
3. Autogenous bacterins may be useful in herds where inadequate control is achieved with commercial products.
4. The efficacy of all vaccines depend on adequate milk flow from the sow.

TRANSMISSIBLE GASTROENTERITIS (TGE)

ETIOLOGY: Coronavirus (antigenically similar to FIP virus)

EPIDEMIOLOGY: Occurs in both epizootic and enzootic forms.

A. Epizootic (epidemic or acute TGE)
   1. Pigs of all ages are affected.
   2. Usually occurs in winter.
   3. Occurs when the virus is introduced into a herd with no immunologic experience with the virus.

B. Enzootic (endemic or chronic TGE)
   1. Pigs from 1 to 8 weeks of age are usually affected.
   2. May occur year round with peak incidence in winter.
   3. Occurs in herds that have had experience with the virus—i.e., partial immunity.

C. Transmission
   1. Usually from other infected pigs.
   2. Starlings and dogs may carry and transmit the virus.
   3. Fomites: fecal contamination of boots, clothes, etc.

PATHOGENESIS:

Virus is ingested—infects and destroys small intestinal epithelial cells—atrophy of jejunal villi—derangement of digestion and absorption—undigested lactose may cause osmotic accumulation of fluid in the intestinal lumen → diarrhea and dehydration → metabolic acidosis.

CLINICAL SIGNS:

A. Epizootic (epidemic) form; all ages are affected.
   1. Baby pigs
      a. Vomiting and diarrhea
      b. High morbidity and high mortality in pigs < 2 weeks of age.
      c. Diarrhea may contain curds of undigested milk.
      d. Mortality decreases as age increases.
   2. Growers, finishers, and adults
      a. Anorexia, vomiting, and diarrhea
      b. Sows may be febrile.
      c. Occasional abortions may be observed in pregnant sows.
      d. Usually recover in 7-10 days.

B. Enzootic (endemic) form
   1. Diarrhea is usually not seen before 6-7 days and not after 2 weeks postweaning.
   2. Variable morbidity and mortality but much lower than epizootic form.
   3. Often a component of mixed infections.
   4. Affected pigs may be chronically stunted.
   5. Illness is absent in adults.

DIAGNOSIS:

A. Clinical signs, especially in epizootic form.

B. Gross pathology
   1. Undigested milk in stomach and intestines
   2. Thin walled, nearly transparent intestinal wall
   3. Chyle is absent from mesenteric lymphatics.

C. Histopathology: villus atrophy of jejunum

D. Detection of viral antigen: immunofluorescence, ELISA, immune electron microscopy

E. Virus isolation

   Tests for viral antigen and virus isolation are useful in acute cases before infected enterocytes are lost. These tests are often negative in a pig that has been scouring for more than two days.

F. Serology
   1. May be useful to monitor herd status.
   2. A relatively nonpathogenic porcine respiratory coronavirus (PRCV) is

present in some herds and may cause false positives on TGE serology.

E. Fecal pH of < 7 suggests viral (TGE or rota) enteritis.

TREATMENT:

A. None specific
B. Fluid and electrolyte therapy
C. Antibacterial therapy in mixed infections
D. Warm, draft-free, dry environment

PREVENTION AND CONTROL:

A. Management
   1. Do not introduce infected animals.
      a. Although chronic asymptomatic carriers may exist, the vast majority of swine will shed the virus only 2 weeks postinfection. Therefore, isolation of herd additions is important.
      b. Introduce animals from a serologically negative herd. This may be impractical due to the prevalence of false positives from PRCV.
   2. Prevent exposure to starlings and dogs.
   3. Practice sanitation: clean boots, clothing, trucks, etc.
B. Immunization: IgA offers more protection than IgG, therefore mucosal exposure is more effective than parenteral exposure.
   1. Expose sows to virulent virus at least 3 weeks prefarrowing. Feed minced intestines of acutely affected baby pigs to sows or administer gelatin capsule of above material to sows. This material may be frozen at -20°C with no loss of potency.
   2. Commercial modified live virus (MLV) injectable and oral vaccines. All attenuated vaccines seem to be better at boosting immunity than at eliciting a primary immune response.
   3. Oral vaccination of baby piglets
C. Eradication
   1. Recent reports have suggested that eradication of TGE virus from a herd without depopulation is possible. The procedure is based on the assumption that the infected pig does not shed virulent virus longer than 2 weeks.
   2. The basic points of an eradication procedure are:
      a. Close the herd. Any needed replacement animals must be introduced before the eradication procedure begins. The herd will be closed for at least 6 months.
      b. Equalize herd immunity. *All* animals must be dosed with virulent virus. This is done by deliberately infecting susceptible neonates and feeding back intestinal homogenates to other members of the herd.
      c. Strict sanitation and all-in, all-out movement of animals. Eliminate the virus in the environment.
      d. Monitoring. Three months after whole herd dosing, seronegative

sentinel animals are introduced. If these animals remain seronegative after a 30- and 60-day test, successful eradication has likely been accomplished.

Suggested Reading:

Harris DL, BeVier GW, Wiseman BS. 1987. Eradication of transmissible gastroenteritis virus without depopulation. *Proc Am Ass Swine Pract* 555-561.

ROTAVIRAL ENTERITIS

ETIOLOGY: RNA virus—family Reoviridae

EPIDEMIOLOGY:

A. Virus is ubiquitous. Herd infection rates are nearly 100%.
B. Infection is much more prevalent than clinical signs.

PATHOGENESIS:

A. Similar to TGE.
B. Rotavirus is probably synergistic with other enteric pathogens, e.g., *E. coli*, *C. perfringens*, coccidia, and TGE.

CLINICAL SIGNS:

A. Similar to enzootic TGE; usually less severe.
B. Diarrhea almost always occurs 3-4 days following weaning; however, neonatal diarrhea due to rotavirus is occasionally reported.
C. Mortality is low; morbidity is variable.
D. Associated with poor doing nursery pigs, i.e., "failure to bloom."

DIAGNOSIS: Can be difficult.

A. History and clinical signs
B. Gross pathology
   1. Thin-walled intestine
   2. Poorly digested food material in the intestine
C. Histopathology: villus atrophy (duodenum is *not* spared as in TGE).
D. Fluorescent antibody
E. Electron microscopy
F. Other enteric pathogens are often found in association with rotavirus.

TREATMENT:

A. Glucose and electrolytes orally
B. Antibacterials for concurrent *E. coli*

PREVENTION AND CONTROL:

A. Weaning management
    1. Wean pigs into a clean, warm, dry, draft-free environment.
    2. Insure good nutritional management.
    3. Control concurrent disease.
B. Vaccination.
    1. Orally administered modified live virus (MLV) vaccines at 7 and 21 days or via drinking water at weaning have shown some benefit.
    2. Heterogeneity of strains may hamper vaccination success.

COCCIDIOSIS

HISTORY: Coccidial infections have been known to exist in swine since 1878; it has been recognized as a clinical problem only since 1975.

ETIOLOGY: *Isospora suis*. Many species of *Eimeria* and *Isospora* are found in swine; however, only *I. suis* is commonly associated with clinical disease.

EPIDEMIOLOGY:

A. Coccidial infections are a component of up to 27% of 5 day to weaning diarrheas.
B. The major source of infective oocysts is scouring baby pigs. Sows shed *I. suis* infrequently if at all.
C. Coccidiosis is more of a problem in systems with continuous farrowing and poor sanitation.
D. Mixed infections (especially with *E. coli*) are common.

PATHOGENESIS:

Sporulated oocysts are ingested—sporozoites invade intestinal epithelial cells and become trophozoites—these divide and form meronts or schizonts—each meront or schizont gives rise to many merozoites which are released from (thus destroying) the host cell—merozoites invade other epithelial cells and either repeat the cycle or become gametes—gametes fuse to form oocysts, are released from the cell (destroying it) and pass in the feces where they sporulate. Destruction of enterocytes (primarily villus epithelium of the jejunum and ileum) results in primarily a malabsorptive diarrhea.

CLINICAL SIGNS:

A. Diarrhea
   1. Usually begins between 7 and 10 days of age.
   2. Yellow to gray-green watery feces
   3. *Not* bloody (in contrast to calves)
   4. Usually acidic pH
   5. Unresponsive to most antimicrobial therapy.

B. Gauntness and dehydration

C. Variable morbidity and mortality
   1. Often increases in time.
   2. May be influenced by concurrent bacterial and viral infections.

DIAGNOSIS:

A. Clinical signs: especially the age of pigs affected. Diarrheas in pigs less than 7 days of age are not due to coccidiosis.

B. Fecal flotation may be misleading. Oocysts are often absent from diarrhetic feces.
   1. Oocyst excretion is biphasic: 5-8 days postinfection (p.i.) and 11-14 days p.i.
   2. Diarrhea usually occurs 8-10 days p.i.

C. Necropsy
   1. Mild to severe fibrinonecrotic enteritis
   2. Usually limited to jejunum and ileum.

D. Histopathology
   1. Villus atrophy
   2. Variable amounts of ulceration and necrosis of the intestinal mucosa
   3. Coccidial forms (merozoites) seen in epithelial cells.

E. Impression smears and demonstration of merozoites

TREATMENT:

A. No coccidiostats are approved for use in swine. All treatment regimes discussed below are extra-label uses. Appropriate guidelines and precautions must be followed.

B. Sow treatment
   1. Coccidiostats approved for cattle (decoquinate, amprolium) have been fed to sows and will decrease fecal shedding of coccidial oocysts. However, since the coccidia in sows are usually nonpathogenic *Eimeria* spp., this

practice is of no clinical benefit.
2. The FDA does not consider the use of feed additives in an off-label manner to be an acceptable extra-label drug use. The addition of coccidiostats to sow feed is not only useless but also illegal.

B. Pig treatment
1. 2 ml of 9.6% amprolium solution orally for 3 days
2. Oral trimethoprim/sulfa
3. Pig treatments are labor-intensive and of limited efficacy.

PREVENTION AND CONTROL:

A. Practice all-in, all-out farrowing house management.
B. Clean thoroughly and disinfect with 5% Clorox.
C. Change to raised farrowing crates with woven wire or expanded metal flooring.

CLOSTRIDIAL ENTERITIS

ETIOLOGY: *Clostridium perfringens* type C

EPIDEMIOLOGY:

A. Most commonly occurs in first 3-4 days of life, though it occasionally occurs in weaned pigs.
B. Mortality varies greatly from herd to herd (0-100%); mortality of affected pigs varies according to age (greater in younger pigs).
C. Sow probably carries the organism in feces and on skin; pig is inoculated soon after birth.
D. The organism can become established in the soil.

PATHOGENESIS:

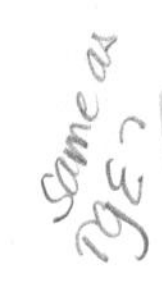

Piglets consume organism shortly after birth—organism attaches to and invades jejunal villi—elaboration of beta (and other) toxins contribute to massive intestinal necrosis—death results from secondary bacteremia, hypoglycemia, and toxemia.

CLINICAL SIGNS:

A. Peracute
1. Sudden death in 1- to 2-day-old piglets
2. May or may not see bloody diarrhea.

B. Acute
1. 2- to 3-day course usually resulting in death

   2. Bloody diarrhea with shreds of necrotic mucosa

C. Subacute
   1. 5- to 7-day course
   2. Diarrhea may or may not be bloody.
   3. Pigs gradually waste away; progressive emaciation and dehydration.

D. Chronic
   1. Intermittent diarrhea
   2. Variable mortality; survivors are chronically stunted.
   3. Some believe these pigs to be more susceptible to hemorrhagic bowel syndrome later in life.

DIAGNOSIS:

A. Clinical signs. Hemorrhagic diarrhea in nursing piglets is very suggestive of clostridial enteritis.

B. Lesions
   1. Bloody fluid in jejunum and occasionally neighboring regions of the intestine
   2. Necrotic membrane in the lumen of the jejunum with variable amounts of hemorrhage
   3. Emphysema in jejunal submucosa
   4. Large gram positive rods lining the jejunal mucosa may be seen microscopically in peracute and acute cases.
   5. Chronic cases show a necrotic enteritis that is difficult to distinguish from other chronic enteropathies, especially coccidiosis.
   6. Demonstration of *C. perfringens* type C beta toxin in intestinal fluid is diagnostic but usually unnecessary.
   7. Isolation of organism is suggestive but not pathognomonic.

TREATMENT:

A. Usually ineffective once clinical signs are evident.

B. Administration of type C antitoxin may help in acute and subacute cases.

PREVENTION AND CONTROL:

A. Sanitation: wash the sow to remove organisms from her skin and udder before moving her into the farrowing house.

B. Parenteral and/or oral administration of type C antitoxin within minutes of birth may be protective. Give 2 ml orally and 2 ml subcutaneously.

C. Vaccination of sow with *C. perfringens* type C toxoid 5 and 2 weeks before farrowing.

D. Prophylactic antibiotics
   1. Bacitracin (BMD)
      a. 250 g/ton BMD in sow feed 2 weeks prior to farrowing and through

3 weeks of lactation

b. Add BMD to peat moss-based oral iron to give each piglet 10 mg/day from day 4-5 to 3 weeks (50 g per 12.5 pound bag; one-half ounce per pig per day).

2. Virginiamycin (Stafac)—extra-label

a. 50 g/ton Stafac in sow feed 2 weeks prior to farrowing and through lactation

b. 10 g Stafac per 12.5 pound bag of peat moss-based oral iron; feed at one-half ounce per pig per day.

3. Prophylactic doses of penicillin or amoxicillin (oral or parenteral) given to piglets at birth.

POSTWEANING SCOURS

GENERAL:

A. In nature, weaning is a gradual process of dietary change from milk to solid food; it may not be complete until the pig is 10 to 12 weeks of age.

B. In modern swine production, weaning is a sudden removal of the pig from the sow which may occur as early as 1 to 3 weeks of age.

C. The 3-week-old pig has an immature digestive system (adapted to digest lactose, milk protein, and fat rather than starches, other sugars, and plant protein) and an immature thermoregulatory system. This pig's immunity is likely at its lowest level (waning colostral immunity, developing active immunity). This pig is highly susceptible to social stress (removal from the dam, mixing and moving with other pigs).

D. Other than parturition, weaning is the most critical and stressful transition in a pig's life.

ETIOLOGY:

A. Diarrhea may occur just from dietary changes at weaning in the absence of any pathogenic agent.

B. More often than not, one or more pathogenic agents can be isolated from cases of postweaning scours.

1. The most common isolates are hemolytic *E. coli*, rotavirus, and TGE.

2. Other occasional isolates are coccidia, *Clostridium*, *Salmonella*, *Campylobacter*, *Serpulina hyodysenteriae*, and others.

C. The stresses of weaning make the pig more susceptible to any of these pathogens.

EPIDEMIOLOGY:

A. Many pigs will scour to some degree postweaning. Depending on the severity, this may or may not be of clinical or economic significance.
B. Many of the more severe cases are associated with some deficiencies of management, e.g., nutrition, environment, sanitation.

PATHOGENESIS:

Frequently, the newly weaned pig goes off feed for the first few days postweaning. Eventually hunger prevails and/or the pig figures out where the food is and what it is for and engorges itself. Immature digestive enzymes leave sugars and starches undigested in the gut lumen. This may cause an osmotic gradient drawing water into the gut. Undigested food may provide a substrate for pathogenic bacteria. Decreased gastric acidity may allow pathogens that would otherwise be killed in the stomach to pass through to the small intestine. Mild villous atrophy with decreased absorptive capacity of the intestine may result from dietary changes at weaning. Decreased immune status may allow pathogens to proliferate. Pathogenic mechanisms of specific pathogenic agents (e.g., *E. coli*, rotavirus) are discussed elsewhere.

CLINICAL SIGNS:

A. Diarrhea which occurs within 1 week after weaning
B. Variable morbidity and mortality depending on the etiology

DIAGNOSIS: Covered in other sections of the outline related to specific etiologies. Diagnostic failures and multiple diagnoses are common.

TREATMENT:

A. Depends on the specific diagnosis.
B. Antimicrobial drugs administered through feed or water are usually indicated, e.g., apramycin, gentamicin, neomycin.
C. Oral glucose and electrolytes for dehydration
D. Water acidifiers (e.g., Bluelite)

PREVENTION AND CONTROL:

A. Weaning management
  1. Later weaning will decrease sow productivity and may complicate pig flow through facilities but this may be the most practical solution for some farms.
  2. All-in, all-out nursery management allows for improved sanitation.
  3. Environmental management: prevent chilling, drafts, etc.
  4. Split weaning: wean larger pigs first, allow small pigs to catch up for a

few days before weaning them. (Rule of thumb—wean only pigs weighing over 12 pounds.)

5. Keeping litters together during the early postweaning period may reduce social stress.

B. Nutritional management
   1. Creep feeding: allow preweaned pigs access to the nursery ration; this gets them used to eating solid feed and may induce digestive enzyme development.
   2. Quality nursery ration: use a high quality, high milk product commercial nursery ration for at least the first few days postweaning; this is more digestible than corn-soybean meal rations.
   3. Feed the newly weaned pig small amounts frequently, i.e., 4 or more times daily. If the pig does not clean up all the feed between feedings, remove the old feed; do not allow it to get stale. In short, do not allow the pig to get into a negative energy balance.

C. Immunization
   1. Depends on the etiology.
   2. Rotavirus and TGE vaccination are discussed in those sections of the outline.
   3. In general, sow vaccination for *E. coli* is not efficacious against postweaning strains of *E. coli*.

Suggested Reading:

van Beers-Schreurs HMG, Vellenga L, Wensing T, and Breukink HJ. 1992. The pathogenesis of the post-weaning syndrome in weaned piglets; a review. *Vet Q* 14:29-34.

SWINE DYSENTERY

ETIOLOGY: *Serpulina (Treponema) hyodysenteriae*

EPIDEMIOLOGY:

A. Clinical disease usually occurs in growing and finishing swine. Morbidity in affected, untreated herds is high (up to 90%); mortality is up to 30%.

B. The organism is primarily transmitted from pig to pig by fecal-oral route. Asymptomatic carrier pigs are common. The organism may also be carried by mice (reservoir host), dogs, birds, rats, and flies (mechanical hosts). Humans may also transmit via fomites.

C. The organism may survive longer than 60 days in manure pits and lagoons. Mice may carry the organism for more than 200 days.

PATHOGENESIS:

S. hyodysenteriae is ingested with contaminated fecal material—it attaches to and invades the colonic mucosa (probably with the help of normal anaerobic flora)—it deranges colonic reabsorptive capacity (unknown mechanism) and produces a catarrhal hemorrhagic colitis → diarrhea and dehydration.

CLINICAL SIGNS:

A. Diarrhea
   1. Usually begins as yellow to gray soft feces.
   2. Later, feces contain large amounts of mucus and sometimes flecks of blood.
   3. Progresses to watery mixture of blood, mucus, and shreds of white mucofibrinous exudate.
B. Anorexia and fever may occur.
C. Thirst due to dehydration.
D. Pigs become gaunt, weak, and emaciated.
E. Most pigs recover in 2 weeks (may be chronic poor doers) but up to 30% may die.
F. Pigs that have recovered from swine dysentery (SD) may be partially immune. Treatment with some drugs inhibits an immune response.
G. Occasionally peracute deaths are seen.
H. Clinical signs of SD may recur within a herd at 3- to 4-week intervals.

DIAGNOSIS:

An accurate diagnosis is essential. Diseases that can be confused with SD include:
   1. Whipworms
   2. Salmonellosis
   3. Proliferative enteropathy (ileitis)
   4. Gastric ulcers
   5. Hemorrhagic bowel syndrome

A. Clinical signs
B. Gross lesions
   1. Mucohemorrhagic colitis. Pseudomembranes are occasionally present. Lesions are typically absent from the small intestine.
   2. Hyperemia and edema of the walls and mesentery of the large intestine
C. Microscopic lesions
   1. Thickened colonic mucosa and submucosa
   2. Hyperplasia of goblet cells
   3. Hemorrhage and superficial necrosis of mucosa

4. Accumulations of fibrin, mucus, and cellular debris

D. Observation of organism
   1. Darkfield examination of mucosal smears
   2. Gram's or Victoria blue 4R stained mucosal scrapings
   3. Silver stained histologic sections
   4. For diagnostic techniques involving direct observation of the organism, large numbers of spirochetes must be demonstrated as small numbers of nonpathogenic spirochetes may be present in normal animals.

E. Culture
   1. Definitive diagnostic test
   2. Requires specialized techniques; check with lab.
   3. Should be acutely affected, unmedicated pig.
   4. Fecal cultures are not reliable for detecting carrier animals.

F. Serologic tests have been described but are not widely used.

TREATMENT:

Many antimicrobial drugs are reported to have some activity against SD. The causative organism has apparently developed resistance to many of them. Drugs presented here are administered via either feed or water. Water medication is probably the route of choice in an acute outbreak.

A. Carbadox (Mecadox—Pfizer)
   1. Mix in feed at 50 g/ton
   2. Must not be fed to pigs over 75 pounds nor within 10 weeks of slaughter.

B. Lincomycin (Lincomix—Upjohn)
   1. Mix in water at 250 mg/gallon (one pkg per 64 gallons). Give for 5 days after bloody stools disappear but for no more than 10 consecutive days.
   2. Mix in feed at 100 g/ton and feed for 3 weeks for treatment followed by 40 g/ton to market weight for control.
   3. Withdrawal time for 100 g/ton level is 6 days; no withdrawal is required at the 40 g/ton level.

C. Tiamulin (Denagard—Fermenta)
   1. Mix in drinking water at concentration to provide 3.5 mg per pound body weight. Give for 5 days. Withdraw 3 days prior to slaughter.
   2. Mix in feed at 35 g/ton. Withdraw 2 days prior to slaughter.

D. Gentamicin (Garacin—Schering)
   1. Mix in water at 50 mg/gallon, 3-day treatment.
   2. Ten-day withdrawal time

E. Bacitracin methylene disalicylate (BMD—A.L. Labs)
   1. Mix in feed at 250 g/ton and feed to slaughter for control.
   2. No withdrawal

F. Other drugs that have been used and may have limited efficacy include:
   1. Arsanilic acid

a. Was at one time the drug of choice.
b. May actually cause carrier pigs to develop clinical disease.
2. Virginiamycin
3. Tylosin
4. Neomycin
5. Oxytetracycline

PREVENTION AND CONTROL:

A. Prevention
1. Ideally, maintain closed herd.
2. If animals must be purchased:
a. Purchase from herds with no known history of SD.
b. Isolate newly purchased stock for 30 days.
c. Medicate newly purchased stock.

B. Vaccination
1. *Serpulina hyodysenteriae* is a poor immunogen.
2. Currently, one federally licensed vaccine is available (Hy-Guard—Haver).
a. Will not prevent infection, clinical signs, or carriers.
b. May reduce severity of clinical signs.

C. Eradication of disease in infected herds
1. Depopulation, clean-up, disinfection, and repopulation with *S. hyodysenteriae*-free stock.
2. Medication and sanitation
a. Carbadox, lincomycin, and tiamulin have been utilized in successful eradication programs. Medicate *every* pig on the farm for at least 4 to 6 weeks. Observe appropriate withdrawal times.
b. Sanitation: *thoroughly* clean and disinfect facilities. Drain and clean pits. Do not recycle lagoon water during clean-up. Empty dirt lots, disk ground, and allow to dry in warm sunlight before using again.
c. Eliminate rodents. Use professional exterminators.
d. After completion of medication and sanitation, discontinue use of drugs or vaccines to suppress swine dysentery. Observe herd for clinical signs. Successful eradication is presumed if no clinical signs are observed for 6 months after vaccines and drugs have been discontinued.

Suggested Reading:

Swine Dysentery—Practitioner Planning Guide for Herd Elimination Programs. Livestock Conservation Institute, 1990; 16pp. (available from the AASP)

PROLIFERATIVE ENTEROPATHY

SYNONYMS: Porcine intestinal adenomatosis
Regional ileitis
Terminal ileitis
Necrotic enteritis
Proliferative hemorrhagic enteropathy
"Garden hose gut"

Hemorrhagic bowel syndrome is distinct from above in clinical presentation and probably in etiology; it is discussed separately.

ETIOLOGY:

A. *Ileobacter intracellularis* is the proposed name of a newly discovered obligate intracellular bacterium believed to cause this disease. The organism is also referred to as ileal symbiont intracellularis.
B. Because these organisms morphologically resemble *Campylobacter* species, this was previously thought to be a part of the etiology. However, the disease cannot be reproduced with *Campylobacter* species.

EPIDEMIOLOGY:

A. Little is known.
B. Subclinical disease is probably widespread.
C. Disease may be more apparent in SPF (specific-pathogen-free) or minimal disease herds.
D. Usually occurs in the grower/finisher period but may occur at any age.
E. May be induced by stress (weaning, movement, weather, etc.).
F. May be genetic predisposition.

PATHOGENESIS: Poorly understood.

CLINICAL SIGNS:

A. May be mild or inapparent; reduced feed intake and growth rate.
B. Intermittent diarrhea; anorexia and weight loss; variable morbidity, mortality usually low.
C. Melena, hemorrhagic diarrhea (more common in older pigs), occasional acute deaths but most recover.
D. Anemia

DIAGNOSIS:

A. Clinical signs are vague. May be confused with almost any other enteric disease of swine.
B. Gross lesions
   1. Thickened intestinal mucosa ("garden hose gut").
   2. May be variable amounts of ulceration, necrosis and hemorrhage. Fibrinonecrotic pseudomembranes may be present.
   3. Lesions are usually limited to the distal third of the small intestine, cecum, and proximal third of the spiral colon.
C. Histopathology
   1. Proliferation of intestinal epithelial glands
   2. See B.2. above.
   3. Small, curved, intracellular organisms in the cytoplasm of proliferating cells can be demonstrated with silver stains.
D. DNA probes. Hybridization of fecal extracts with DNA probes specific for *Ileobacter intracellularis* is the most specific diagnostic test.

TREATMENT:

A. Treatment should be thought of as preventive rather than curative. Occasionally individual animals will respond to injectable antibiotics (tylosin).
B. Positive prophylactic effects have been reported with a wide variety of feed and water medications, i.e., tylosin, neomycin, carbadox, tetracyclines, penicillin, bacitracin, copper sulfate.

PREVENTION AND CONTROL:

A. Reduce stress.
B. Medicate at times of unavoidable stress.
C. Genetic selection (questionable)

HEMORRHAGIC BOWEL SYNDROME

DEFINITION: An acute, fatal disease of swine characterized by massive hemorrhage into the intestines without evidence of ulceration, torsion, or volvulus.

ETIOLOGY: Unknown. Some theories include:

A. A peracute form of proliferative enteropathy
B. Hypersensitivity to milk protein ("whey bloat"), *E. coli* toxins, or mycotoxins

C. Endotoxic shock
D. A late form of clostridial enteritis

EPIDEMIOLOGY:

A. Sporadic, low morbidity (1-2%)
B. Usually occurs in growers or finishers.
C. May see higher incidence in times of stress.

CLINICAL SIGNS:

A. Acute death
B. Pale carcass that bloats rapidly

DIAGNOSIS:

A. Thin walled, dark red intestine with massive amounts of blood in the lumen
B. No evidence of gastric ulceration, intestinal torsion, salmonellosis, swine dysentery, or proliferative enteritis.
C. May see large numbers of eosinophils in the lamina propria on histologic examination.

TREATMENT: One report indicates a reduction in death losses after adding 100 g/ton chlortetracycline and 50 g/ton bacitracin (BMD) to the feed.

WHIPWORMS

ETIOLOGY: *Trichuris suis*

EPIDEMIOLOGY:

A. Clinical disease occurs most commonly at 2-6 months of age.
B. Ova are very resistant.
C. Life cycle
    1. Eggs are passed in feces and require at least 3 weeks to become infective.
    2. Eggs are ingested and hatch in the small intestine and cecum.
    3. Larvae develop in the mucosa of the cecum for 2 weeks (histotrophic phase).
    4. The posterior segment of the worm develops into the lumen while the thin anterior segment remains embedded in the mucosa.
    5. Prepatency is 41-47 days; longevity is 4-5 months.

PATHOGENESIS:

A. *Trichuris suis* interacts with other secondary bacterial invaders (usually spirochetes but not necessarily *S. hyodysenteriae*) to cause a catarrhal enteritis.
B. Infection of SPF or gnotobiotic pigs results in no clinical signs and very little pathology.

CLINICAL SIGNS:

A. Diarrhea with mucus and blood
B. Dehydration and emaciation
C. Anorexia
D. Anemia
E. Occasional deaths

DIAGNOSIS: Must be differentiated from other hemorrhagic diarrheas of growing swine, especially swine dysentery.

A. Clinical signs
B. Fecal flotation; ova are shed sporadically.
C. Necropsy
   1. Catarrhal enteritis, fibrinonecrotic membranes in large intestine
   2. Demonstration of worms
D. Response to therapy

TREATMENT:

A. Effective anthelmintics include dichlorvos (Atgard) and fenbendazole (Safe-guard).
B. Ivermectin is *not* very efficacious against whipworms.

PREVENTION AND CONTROL:

A. Sanitation
B. Anthelmintics

GASTRIC ULCERS

ETIOLOGY: Speculative. Risk factors include:

A. Finely ground feed. Feed particles less than 350 μm in diameter are ulcerogenic.
B. Stresses associated with shipment, e.g., withholding of feed.

C. Other factors that may increase the risk of gastric ulceration include selenium and/or vitamin E deficiency, copper toxicity and/or zinc deficiency, Vitamin U (methylmethionine-sulfonium) deficiency.

EPIDEMIOLOGY: Usually sporadic, low morbidity

PATHOGENESIS: Speculative. Supposedly an increase in gastric acidity is necessary for the development of gastric ulcers. The mechanisms that produce this are not well understood.

CLINICAL SIGNS:

A. Anorexia and depression
B. Anemia due to gastric hemorrhage
C. May see melena.
D. Occasional sudden deaths due to exsanguination

DIAGNOSIS:

A. Antemortem diagnosis may be difficult.
B. Lesions
   1. Ulceration of the squamous gastric epithelium
   2. Parakeratosis is considered a preulcerative lesion.

TREATMENT: Usually unrewarding

A. Antacids: aluminum hydroxide, magnesium silicate
B. Vitamin E and selenium
C. Reduce stress, put out on pasture (a possible source of vitamin U).

PREVENTION AND CONTROL:

A. Coarsely ground feed; use >3.5 mm screen size.
B. Selenium supplementation
C. If copper is added to feed, 110 ppm zinc carbonate should also be added.
D. Reduce stress

5

CENTRAL NERVOUS SYSTEM DISEASES

MYOCLONIA CONGENITA

SYNONYMS: Congenital tremors, shaker pigs, dancing pig disease

ETIOLOGY: Congenital tremors virus (CTV). Other heritable, infectious (hog cholera, pseudorabies), and toxic (trichlorfon) etiologies of congenital tremors have been described; however, CTV is the most common.

EPIDEMIOLOGY:

A. Virus spreads laterally among mature pigs with no clinical signs; effects are seen only in baby pigs.
B. Boars may chronically shed virus and infect female at breeding.
C. Usually affects entire litter.
D. Sows will usually have only one affected litter. Subsequent litters will be normal.

PATHOGENESIS:

A. Virus infects fetuses in late gestation.
B. Virus retards normal myelin deposition.

CLINICAL SIGNS:

A. Varying severity of tremors of head and limbs of neonatal piglets
B. Tremors subside as piglet sleeps.
C. Variable mortality: if the piglet can nurse, it will probably live.

D. Piglets that survive gradually improve.

DIAGNOSIS:

A. Obvious from clinical signs.
B. Necropsy: decreased myelin content in spinal cord.
C. May want to rule out other causes, especially PRV and trichlorfon toxicity.

TREATMENT: None specific. Supportive therapy may reduce mortality.

PREVENTION AND CONTROL:

A. Incidence within a herd will usually spontaneously decrease as more females become immune.
B. Herd additions (especially purchased gilts) should be exposed to endemic herd pathogens before breeding.
C. Other questionable recommendations include culling the boar that has sired an affected litter (of little benefit unless etiology is heritable), and not saving boars from affected litters (may be chronic carriers).

NEONATAL HYPOGLYCEMIA

ETIOLOGY:

A. Inadequate intake of milk
  1. Lactation failure of sow
  2. Illness or defect of piglet
B. Low environmental temperatures may exacerbate.

PATHOGENESIS:

A. The newborn piglet has limited glycogen and body fat stores.
B. Fasting gluconeogenesis is not efficient until the pig is >6-7 days of age.
C. The piglet is dependent on a steady supply of milk to maintain normal (80-100 mg/dl) blood glucose.
D. As blood glucose falls below 50 mg/dl, clinical signs may develop.

CLINICAL SIGNS:

A. Seen in piglets < 7 days of age
B. Uncertain gait, convulsions, shivering, hypothermia
C. Death usually occurs within 24-36 hours of the onset of clinical signs.

DIAGNOSIS:

A. Blood glucose <50 mg/dl (may be as low as 7 mg/dl)
B. May have empty stomachs

TREATMENT:

A. If the pig is severely depressed or comatose, inject 1 to 2 g of glucose per kg body weight (20 ml/kg of warm 5% glucose solution injected intraperitoneally).
B. As hypoglycemic pigs are usually hypothermic as well, they should be gradually warmed to 102°F (39°C).
C. After the pig regains normal CNS function, energy intake should be sustained via oral nutritional supplementation. Milk replacer or commercial nutritional supplements should be given.

PREVENTION AND CONTROL:

Correct the primary cause of inadequate milk flow or milk intake.

STREPTOCOCCAL MENINGITIS

ETIOLOGY: *Streptococcus* spp., especially *Streptococcus suis* type II

EPIDEMIOLOGY:

A. Subclinical carriers are common. The organism can be frequently cultured from the tonsillar crypts of clinically normal pigs.
B. The organism is transmitted via respiratory route—contact and aerosols.
C. Stress (e.g., crowding, poor ventilation) may precipitate an outbreak.
D. Concurrent infections—e.g., pseudorabies, porcine reproductive and respiratory syndrome (PRRS), *Bordetella bronchiseptica*—can intensify disease resulting from infection with *Streptococcus suis*.
E. While this organism is often isolated from pneumonic lungs, its role as a respiratory pathogen is not well established. Usually other respiratory pathogens can also be isolated from these lungs.
F. *Strep. suis* is *not* usually eliminated from a herd by minimal disease technologies such as SPF or segregated early weaning. Pigs from minimal disease herds may be *more* susceptible to disease than conventional pigs.
G. Two virulence markers have been identified. One is a cell-wall associated protein known as muramidase-released-protein (MRP); the other is known as extracellular factor (EF).
    1. MRP+ EF+ strains are most virulent.

2. MRP+ EF- strains are of intermediate virulence.
3. MRP- EF- strains are nonvirulent.

PATHOGENESIS:

A. Organism colonizes tonsils—is phagocytized by monocytes—travels via monocytes through the general circulation to the cerebrospinal fluid (CSF) and meninges—there an inflammatory response causes increased pressure in the CSF, which results in neurologic signs.
B. Although the relationship of virulence markers to pathogenesis is not well understood, it is believed that pathogenic strains are better able to survive phagocytosis by macrophages than are nonpathogenic strains.

CLINICAL SIGNS:

A. Usually occurs 3-12 weeks of age.
B. Morbidity usually low but up to 50%; mortality up to 50%.
C. Fever, anorexia, depression, tremors, blindness, ataxia, convulsions, death

DIAGNOSIS:

A. Clinical signs
B. Lesions
    1. Congestion and edema of brain and meninges
    2. Suppurative meningitis
    3. Polyserositis
C. Culture of CSF or meningeal swab

TREATMENT:

A. Penicillin, ampicillin, streptomycin, tetracyclines
B. Antiserum (Suis Serum—Grand Laboratories)
C. Must be initiated early.

PREVENTION AND CONTROL:

A. Minimize stress
B. Prophylactic antibiotics
C. Commercial whole cell bacterins are available and are reasonably efficacious.

NOTE: *Streptococcus suis* type II may infect humans. While infection is unusual, it has been identified as an occupational disease of slaughterhouse workers, farm workers, and veterinarians. Clinical signs include meningitis, deafness, dizziness, and recurring headaches. Be careful when working with infected pigs and tissues.

Suggested Reading:

Chanter N, Jones PW, and Alexander TJL. 1993. Meningitis in pigs caused by *Streptococcus suis*—a speculative review. *Vet Microbiol* 36:39-55.
Pijoan C. 1994. Diagnosis of *Streptococcus suis* infections. *Swine Health and Prod* 2(4):19-20.

SALT POISONING

SYNONYMS: Sodium ion (Na^+) toxicity, water deprivation

ETIOLOGY:

A. Direct salt poisoning—consumption of excess Na^+ —uncommon.
   1. Excess salt in ration—mixing mistake
   2. Access to brine
   3. Feeding milk by-products (e.g., whey with a high Na^+ content)
B. Indirect salt poisoning—water deprivation followed by water intoxication—much more common than direct salt poisoning. Water deprivation may be due to:
   1. Frozen water
   2. Malfunctioning automatic waterers
   3. Insufficient waterer space
   4. Management mistakes, e.g., forgetting to turn water back on after making plumbing repairs.
   5. Medicated water unpalatable

PATHOGENESIS: Water deprivation causes a hyperosmolarity of the CNS; as water is consumed, the osmotic pressure draws water into the CNS causing swelling and edema of the brain.

CLINICAL SIGNS:

A. Thirst, constipation, restlessness
B. Depression, blindness, deafness, convulsions, death

DIAGNOSIS:

A. Clinical signs
B. History of water deprivation or high salt diet
C. Clinical pathology: hemoconcentration, eosinopenia, hypernatremia, hyperchloremia

D. Lesions
   1. Meningoencephalitis with edema
   2. Eosinophilic perivascular cuffing in cerebral cortex and meninges—pathognomonic

TREATMENT: Generally ineffectual

PREVENTION AND CONTROL:

A. Provide free access to water.
   1. Adequate supply, not frozen, etc.
   2. Be sure pigs can operate automatic waterers.
B. Reduce salt in feed and water; <1% in feed; <0.5% in water.

EDEMA DISEASE

ETIOLOGY:

A. Certain serotypes of *E. coli* that produce a specific toxin.
B. Serotypes commonly associated with edema disease include O138:K81, O139:K82, O141:K85. Note that these are not the same strains commonly associated with neonatal colibacillosis.
C. Edema disease strains of *E. coli* are also usually hemolytic.

EPIDEMIOLOGY:

A. Usually occurs from 1 to 3 weeks after weaning. This coincides with the waning of passive immunity that the pig has obtained through colostrum and milk.
B. Other stresses of weaning, such as changes in diet and variations in environmental temperature, may predispose a pig to edema disease.
C. Some pigs are naturally resistant to infection and disease from edema-disease-producing strains of *E. coli*. This is thought to be genetically controlled. Presumably, resistant pigs lack receptors for either the adhesin or the toxin associated with edema disease.
D. Morbidity is usually low, case mortality rate is very high (up to 100%).

PATHOGENESIS:

A. Colonization. Edema disease strains of *E. coli* must adhere to the intestine via fimbria or other adhesion factors. Fimbrial type F107 is commonly associated with edema disease strains of *E. coli*.
B. Toxin

1. Edema-disease strains of *E. coli* produce a toxin known as Shiga-like toxin type II variant (SLT-IIv). This toxin has also been called edema disease principle (EDP).
2. The toxin is absorbed from the intestinal lumen into the general circulation.
3. The toxin binds to certain receptors on target cells and inhibits cellular protein synthesis. Metabolic functions of the cell are compromised.
4. Some vascular endothelial cells are apparently susceptible to the effects of the toxin. Vascular injury results in edema in various tissues.

CLINICAL SIGNS:

A. May see sudden death with no clinical signs.
B. Anorexia, ataxia, convulsions, palpebral (eyelid) edema, "squeaky" squeal, constipation and/or diarrhea, death within 24 hours.

DIAGNOSIS:

A. Clinical signs: especially palpebral edema
B. Necropsy: widespread edema—subcutaneous, submucosa of stomach along the greater curvature, spiral colon, brain
C. Histopath: segmental necrosis of myocytes in the tunica media of small arteries and arterioles
D. Culture
   1. Isolation of hemolytic *E. coli* from the small intestine and colon, often in pure culture.
   2. Detection of toxin production
      a. By cytotoxicity in Vero cell culture
      b. By DNA probes for toxin

TREATMENT: Ineffective if clinical signs have developed.

PREVENTION AND CONTROL:

A. Antibiotics in feed or water; apramycin, others.
B. Restricted feeding, small frequent feedings
C. Creep feeding
D. High fiber diets
E. Immunization. Although experimental vaccination with a SLT-IIv toxoid has been reported as efficacious, no commercial vaccines are available.

Suggested Reading:

Imberechts H, DeGreve H, and Lintermans P. 1992. The pathogenesis of edema disease in pigs. A review. *Vet Microbiol* 31:221-233.

6

MUSCULOSKELETAL DISEASES

NEONATAL POLYARTHRITIS

ETIOLOGY:

A. Infectious factors. Streptococci, especially group C (*Streptococcus equisimilis*) and group L, are the most common isolates. Staphylococci, *E. coli*, and *Actinomyces (Corynebacterium) pyogenes* are also isolated.
B. Host factors: neonatal polyarthritis seems to be associated with low levels of colostral immunity.
   1. Occurs more often in litters of low parity sows.
   2. May occur more often in poor milking sows.
C. Other factors (management, environment, etc.)
   1. The causative organisms are common in the environment.
   2. Organisms gain entrance via breaks in the skin or mucus membranes.
      a. Umbilical infections
      b. Tail docking, ear notching, teeth clipping, castration, etc.
      c. Skin (especially carpal) abrasions

PATHOGENESIS:

Organisms enter via breaks in skin or mucus membrane → septicemia → localizes in joints (especially carpus, elbow, hip, hock).

CLINICAL SIGNS:

A. Variable morbidity and mortality (average 3% and 1.5%)
B. Lameness, as early as 3-4 days of age
C. Joint distention, as early as 7-10 days of age
D. May see "fading piglet" syndrome with no clinical lameness.

DIAGNOSIS:

A. Clinical signs
B. Culture
C. Necropsy lesions
   1. Fibrin, pus, and/or necrotic material in the joint capsule
   2. Hyperemia and proliferation of synovial membrane

TREATMENT:

A. Ineffective unless given early
B. Antibiotics according to sensitivity; penicillin, lincomycin, or tylosin are commonly used and usually inhibitory to organisms.

PREVENTION AND CONTROL:

A. Reduce exposure to organisms.
   1. Cleanliness in processing baby pigs
   2. Nonabrasive floor surfaces
   3. Protective carpal covering (Knee-Kote)
   4. Dip navels
B. Improve immunity
   1. Be sure piglets get colostrum.
   2. Farrow older sows.
   3. Antisera for *Streptococcus equisimilis* is commercially available.
C. Prophylactic treatment with antibiotics

SPLAY-LEG

SYNONYMS: Spraddle-leg, myofibrillar hypoplasia

DEFINITION: A congenital defect of piglets characterized by abduction of the hind and/or fore limbs.

ETIOLOGY:

A. Genetic predisposition
B. Slippery floors
C. Nutritional: perhaps choline deficiency
D. Zearalenone ingestion in late gestation

CLINICAL SIGNS:

A. Abduction of limbs; appears within hours of birth.
B. Recovery or death (starvation or crushing) within a week.

DIAGNOSIS:

A. Obvious from clinical signs
B. Pathology: myofibrillar hypoplasia
C. If due to zearalenone, mycotoxin analysis of gestation feed.

TREATMENT: Tape legs together.

PREVENTION AND CONTROL:

A. Genetic selection
B. Provide good footing
C. Choline supplementation of gestation diets at 3-4.5 g per sow daily has been reported to reduce the incidence of splay-leg. Other reports have not confirmed this to be of benefit.
D. Feed gestation rations free of zearalenone.

SUPPURATIVE ARTHRITIS

DEFINITION: A septic arthritis of postweaning pigs characterized by pus in the joint capsules.

ETIOLOGY:

A. *Actinomyces (Corynebacterium) pyogenes* is the most common isolate.
B. Staphylococci and streptococci are occasionally found.
C. All of these organisms are ubiquitous in swine environments.

PATHOGENESIS:

A. Organisms enter via breaks in skin or mucous membrane.
    1. Tail, ear, vulva biting
    2. Contaminated surgical or injection procedures
    3. Lacerations, foot lesions, etc.
    4. Streptococci may enter via tonsil.
B. Become septicemic and localize to joints and other sites (vertebral column, lungs, lymph nodes, etc.).

CLINICAL SIGNS:

A. Lameness
B. Joint distention
C. Abscesses elsewhere on body
D. Usually evidence of cannibalism
E. Chronic poor doers

DIAGNOSIS:

A. Clinical signs
B. Presence of pus in the joint capsule
    1. Detect at necropsy or via arthrocentesis
    2. Color of pus: white and creamy usually indicates strep or staph; yellow or green usually indicates actinomyces.
C. Culture

TREATMENT:

A. Generally unrewarding
B. Antibiotics may be helpful in early stages, i.e., penicillin, lincomycin, tylosin.

PREVENTION & CONTROL: Reduce entry of organisms.

A. Reduce cannibalism.
    1. Reduce crowding.
    2. Reduce group size.
    3. Reduce other social stresses (toys, etc.).
    4. Remove perpetrator.
B. Increase sanitation, especially for injections and surgery.

MYCOPLASMAL ARTHRITIS

ETIOLOGY: *Mycoplasma hyosynoviae*

EPIDEMIOLOGY:

A. Organism is a common nasopharyngeal inhabitant; infected pigs may carry the organism indefinitely.
B. Infection usually occurs between 4 and 12 weeks of age.
C. May see disease in older pigs if animals are moved from an immunologically naive herd (SPF or minimal disease) into a conventional herd (where organism

is endemic).

PATHOGENESIS:

A. Organism infects nasopharynx—becomes septicemic—localizes to joints—especially elbow, stifle, carpus, hock.
B. Not all pigs that have joint infection develop arthritis.
   1. Pigs prone to osteochondrosis may also be prone to mycoplasmal arthritis.
   2. Stress of movement may precipitate arthritis.

CLINICAL SIGNS:

A. Acute or chronic lameness affecting one or more limbs
B. Usually 12-24 weeks of age or 2-5 weeks post movement
C. Usually afebrile and normal appetite
D. +/- joint distention
E. Morbidity variable, mortality very low
F. Cases uncomplicated by osteochondrosis spontaneously improve.

DIAGNOSIS:

A. Clinical signs (unresponsive to penicillin)
B. Necropsy
   1. Serofibrinous to serosanguineous joint fluid (nonsuppurative)
   2. Edematous, hyperemic synovial membranes
C. Culture: should culture acutely diseased, unmedicated pigs; mycoplasmas can be difficult to culture, check with the lab.
D. Serology: complement fixation (CF). This test is not widely available in diagnostic labs and may be of limited use. Many normal pigs have antibody, therefore paired sera must be tested.

TREATMENT:

A. Injectable antibiotics, i.e., lincomycin, tylosin
B. Corticosteroids

PREVENTION & CONTROL:

A. Select for good conformation of breeding stock.
B. Avoid stress of movement.

RICKETS

ETIOLOGY: Deficiency or imbalance of Ca, P, and/or vitamin D

A. Uncommon in modern swine rations
B. May occur due to mixing or formulating errors

PATHOGENESIS:

Ca and P deficiency leads to decreased mineralization of bone.
Vitamin D deficiency leads to decreased deposition of Ca and P into the bony matrix.

CLINICAL SIGNS:

A. Occurs 3-5 months of age
B. Stunted, unthrifty pigs
C. Lame and/or paralyzed pigs due to pathologic fractures.
D. Distorted long bones

DIAGNOSIS:

A. Clinical signs
B. Dietary analysis

NRC recommendations for nursery and finishing hogs

	%Ca	%P	IU/lb feed Vit. D
nursery	0.8	0.6	100
finisher	0.5	0.4	60

C. Necropsy
   1. Enlarged epiphyses
   2. Abnormally shaped diaphyses
   3. "Rachitic rosary" at costochondral junction
   4. Fractures

TREATMENT, PREVENTION, AND CONTROL:

A. Provide adequate levels of Ca, P, and vitamin D in the proper ratio.
B. NRC recommendations are minimum levels for maximum performance; higher levels may be needed for maximum bone strength.

FOOT LESIONS

SYNONYMS: Sore feet, laminitis, foot rot, etc. This is a broad clinical syndrome, not a specific diagnosis.

ETIOLOGY:

A. Trauma to foot
   1. Rough floor finishes
   2. Sharp edges to slat
   3. Narrow slat width
   4. Conformation defects are predisposing factor.
B. Nutritional: biotin deficiency (questionable)
C. Infectious: bacteria may secondarily invade traumatic lesions (bruises, hoof cracks, etc.) leading to septic laminitis (foot rot). *Fusobacterium necrophorum* and *Actinomyces pyogenes* are the most common isolates.

CLINICAL SIGNS:

A. Severe, often unilateral lameness
B. Usually foot lesions are visually apparent. However, not all foot lesions result in lameness. Also, lameness from a traumatic laminitis may exist without visual evidence of a hoof lesion.
C. Palpation elicits painful response.

DIAGNOSIS:

A. Usually obvious from clinical signs.
B. Culture in septic laminitis.
C. Radiology in valuable breeding animals; osteomyelitis indicates a poor prognosis.

TREATMENT: For septic laminitis

A. Penicillin—10,000 IU/lb IM
B. Copper sulfate topically
C. Claw amputation in severe or chronic cases. Prognosis is poor for amputation of lateral claw of a hind limb.

PREVENTION & CONTROL:

A. Improve flooring
   1. Clean, dry, nonabrasive

2. Partial slats vs. total slats
3. "Pencil rounded" edges to slats
4. Wider slats (6"-8" slat; 1" slot)

B. Biotin supplementation—200-400 mg/ton (questionable)
C. Select for soundness.

OSTEOCHONDROSIS

DEFINITIONS:

Osteochondrosis: a disturbance in endochondral ossification.
Osteoarthrosis: degenerative joint disease (DJD), usually secondary to osteochondrosis.
Synonyms and related syndromes:

Osteoarthritis
Osteochondritis dessicans (OCD)
Epiphysitis
DJD
Leg weakness syndrome
Proximal femoral epiphysiolysis
Apophysiolysis of the ischiatic tuberosity

ETIOLOGY:

A. Is *not* infectious.
B. Is correlated with desirable production characteristics, especially rapid growth rate.
  1. Pigs whose feed consumption is restricted by 50% have fewer lesions than full fed swine.
  2. Pigs that have genetically slower growth rates (wild pigs) have fewer lesions than domestic swine.
C. Nutrition probably has no effect, except as it relates to growth rate.
D. Genetics—heritability estimates: 0.30-0.14

EPIDEMIOLOGY:

A. Practically 100% of domestic swine have osteochondrosis.
B. It is not known why some lesions progress to DJD and others heal. Possible factors: conformation, floor surface, stress and trauma to joints.

PATHOGENESIS:

Defects in endochondral ossification occur:

A. Beneath articular cartilage.

may → separation of cartilage from subchondral bone → cartilage flaps or joint mice → chronic degenerative changes in the joint (DJD).

B. At the growth plate.

may → separation of the physis (especially at proximal femur and ischiatic tuberosity).

CLINICAL SIGNS:

A. Osteochondrosis: none.
B. Osteoarthrosis (DJD): chronic, progressive, often bilateral, fore and/or hind leg lameness in an older pig (usually >6 months)
   1. Shortened stride
   2. Carpal flexion
   3. Straight legged, "tip-toe" stance
C. Proximal femoral epiphysiolysis
   1. Acute onset
   2. Down in rear
   3. Bright and alert
   4. Possible crepitus in coxofemoral region
D. Apophysiolysis of the ischiatic tuberosity
   1. Onset: late gestation or early postpartum
   2. "Dog-sitting" posture
   3. Possible crepitus in area of the ischiatic tuberosity

DIAGNOSIS:

A. Clinical signs
B. Radiology
C. Necropsy: presence of lesions of osteochondrosis and/or DJD

TREATMENT:

A. Analgesics (e.g., phenylbutazone, flunixin) may offer symptomatic relief. However, these products are not curative nor are they approved for swine.
B. Conceivably surgical techniques such as those described for dogs and horses could be used; however, these are not considered practical.

PREVENTION AND CONTROL: All of the following are of limited efficacy and/or practicality.

A. Improved floor surfaces may decrease trauma to the joint and decrease the probability that osteochondrosis progresses to osteoarthrosis.
B. Limit feeding to reduce growth rate.
C. Genetic selection

Suggested reading:

Hill MA. 1990. Causes of degenerative joint disease (osteoarthrosis) and dyschondroplasia (osteochondrosis) in pigs. *J Am Vet Med Assoc* 197:107-113.

OSTEOMALACIA

ETIOLOGY: Deficiency or imbalance of Ca, P, and/or vitamin D

PATHOGENESIS:

A. Demand of lactation for Ca and P is not met by dietary intake.
B. Ca and P are mobilized from the bone resulting in reduced mass and strength of bone.

CLINICAL SIGNS:

A. Observed in lactating or recently weaned sows.
B. Acute lameness and/or paralysis, usually affecting the hind limbs
C. May be evidence of fractures; e.g., swelling, crepitus, etc.

DIAGNOSIS:

A. Clinical signs
B. Feed analysis
   National Research Council (NRC) recommendations for lactating sows: 30.0-41.2 g/day Ca; 20.0-27.5 g/day P; 800-1100 IU/day vitamin D. Highly productive sows may need even higher levels.
C. Radiographs: cortical thinning, fractures
D. Necropsy: fractures; histopathology—osteomalacia

TREATMENT: Impractical

PREVENTION AND CONTROL:

A. Provide adequate Ca, P, and vitamin D in the proper ratio. Keep in mind that total intake of Ca, P, and vitamin D is important, not just the percentage in the ration. Factors that limit feed intake in the sow (heat stress, poor palatability of the ration) may lead to deficiencies.
B. Reduce lactational demands—early weaning, cross-fostering.
C. Farrow sows in good condition.
D. Avoid postweaning stress on sows.

PORCINE STRESS SYNDROME (PSS)

SYNONYMS: Malignant hyperthermia (MH); pale, soft, exudative pork (PSE)

ETIOLOGY:

A. Genetic predisposition
   1. Susceptibility to PSS is caused by a single autosomal recessive gene. Disease is manifest only in pigs that are homozygous recessive for this gene.
   2. Caused by a mutation of the ryanodine receptor gene. The protein product of this gene acts as a regulator of Ca^{++} across the cell membrane of muscle cells.
   3. This defective gene seems to be closely associated with positive production characteristics, e.g., good feed conversion, high percent lean. Some have suggested that pigs that are heterozygous for the stress gene are the ideal market hog, i.e., lean but not susceptible to PSS.

B. Stress
   1. Fighting, movement, handling, heat, etc.
   2. Anesthesia. Halothane and other anesthetic agents can induce PSS (usually called malignant hyperthermia in this context).
   3. Poor meat quality (PSE) can result from stresses associated with slaughter (shipment to slaughter; mixing, handling, and moving pigs at the slaughter plant; and during stunning and scalding).

PATHOGENESIS:

The pathophysiological changes that occur during PSS are varied and complex. The following is a basic, possibly oversimplified explanation. The stress-susceptible pig is less able to control Ca^{++} concentration in muscle. Under stress conditions, myoplasmic Ca^{++} concentration increase, causing muscle contraction. As the muscles contract, they produce heat and lactic acid. In severe cases, the body temperature and the lactic acidosis increase to the point of death.

CLINICAL SIGNS: The severity of the clinical signs is related to the degree of stress.

A. Antemortem
   1. Muscle and tail tremors
   2. Dyspnea
   3. Alternating blanched and reddened areas of skin
   4. Increased body temperature
   5. Cyanosis

6. Muscle rigidity
7. Death

B. At slaughter
1. Pale, soft, watery musculature
2. High temperature and low pH leads to protein denaturation and poor quality meat.

DIAGNOSIS: Stress susceptibility is diagnosed by:

A. A DNA probe for the mutant gene. Recently developed, this test can detect both homozygous and heterozygous carrier pigs.

B. Older tests involved exposing a pig to a stressor (e.g., halothane anesthesia, exercise, heat), then checking for the development of clinical signs or muscle damage (elevations of serum creatine phosphokinase [CPK] or pyruvate kinase [PK] levels). These tests will only detect homozygous pigs and have largely given way to the DNA probe test.

TREATMENT:

A. Remove stress.

B. Cool pig down.

C. Dantrolene sodium can block MH.

PREVENTION AND CONTROL:

A. Genetic selection
1. With the DNA probe test, it is possible to eliminate the gene from a population. Some seedstock suppliers are doing this.
2. Other genetic suppliers suggest using heterozygous boars on females free of the stress gene so that some of the offspring will have the lean growth benefits associated with the gene. If this is done, it is imperative that gilts from these matings not be saved for breeding purposes.

B. Avoid excessive stress.

Suggested reading:

Louis CF, Rempel WE, Kennedy CF, Irvin LR, and Mickelson, JR. 1992. The molecular genetic diagnosis of porcine stress syndrome. *AASP Newsletter* 4(3):13-16.

7

REPRODUCTIVE AND UROGENITAL DISEASES

PORCINE PARVOVIRUS (PPV)

ETIOLOGY: Parvoviridae—small DNA virus

EPIDEMIOLOGY:

A. Virus is present in practically 100% of swine herds worldwide.
B. Immune sows provide high levels of passive antibody to nursing piglets.
   1. Passive maternal antibody usually persists for 3-6 months.
   2. Passive maternal antibody effectively prevents infection and active seroconversion.
   3. In unvaccinated herds, active seroconversion usually occurs between 4 and 12 months of age.
C. Virus may be transmitted orally or venereally.
D. A postnatally infected pig may shed the virus for 2 to 3 weeks.
   1. Postnatal infection does not produce persistent carriers.
   2. Prenatal infection (>70 days gestation) may produce immunotolerant, persistent carriers.
E. The virus may survive in the environment for 16 to 20 weeks. It is resistant to many common disinfectants.

PATHOGENESIS:

A. Virus enters susceptible seronegative pig via oronasal route.
B. If male or nonpregnant female, the pig seroconverts and eliminates the virus with no clinical signs.
C. If pregnant female, the virus crosses the placenta and infects rapidly dividing

fetal cells.

1. If conceptus is less than 30 days of age (embryo), it is killed and resorbed by the dam.
2. If conceptus is 30 to 70 days of age (fetus), it is killed and is mummified.
3. If conceptus is greater than 70 days of age (immunocompetent fetus), it mounts an immune response and usually survives to term. The pig may, however, be born dead or weak.
4. The virus usually spreads slowly from fetus to fetus within the uterus.

D. Natural infection probably confers lifetime immunity.

CLINICAL SIGNS:

A. Other than reproductive problems in pregnant females, no signs of illness are observed.
B. Increased normal and delayed returns to estrus
C. Mummified fetuses
   1. Mummies are often different sizes (gestational age) within the same litter.
   2. Mummies may be present with live pigs in the same litter.
D. Small litters
E. Weak and stillborn pigs
F. Abortions are *not* typical of parvovirus infection in swine.
G. This spectrum of clinical signs was at one time called the SMEDI syndrome, for *S*tillbirths, *M*ummified fetuses, *E*mbryonic *D*eath, and *I*nfertility. This syndrome was first associated etiologically with porcine enteroviruses; however, it is now recognized that parvovirus is more frequently the cause.

DIAGNOSIS:

A. Clinical signs
B. Detection of viral antigen in mummified fetuses by immunofluorescent microscopy or hemagglutination
C. Serological demonstration of antibody in dam
   1. Hemagglutination inhibition and serum neutralization tests are used.
   2. Infection is so ubiquitous that a single positive titer is of no help in confirming a diagnosis of reproductive failure due to PPV.

TREATMENT: None

PREVENTION AND CONTROL:

A. Natural infection of gilts before breeding
   1. Commingle gilts with sows before breeding in hopes that some sows will be shedding PPV or that PPV is present in the environment.
   2. Grind up mummified fetuses and feed to gilts before breeding.
   3. If one is successful at inducing a natural infection before breeding, the gilt

should be immune for life; the above methods, however, are not always dependable.

B. Vaccination
   1. Several inactivated vaccines are on the market.
   2. Vaccine immunity lasts from 4 to 6 months, therefore revaccination before every breeding is indicated.
   3. Vaccination delays natural infection and seroconversion, therefore older sows may become susceptible to PPV reproductive failure when vaccine immunity wanes. A low level of sporadic losses due to PPV can be expected even in vaccinated herds.

LEPTOSPIROSIS

ETIOLOGY: *Leptospira interrogans*—many serovars

EPIDEMIOLOGY:

A. Some serovars are host adapted to swine.
   1. *L. pomona* is probably the most common cause of clinical leptospirosis in swine.
   2. *L. bratislava* is common in serologic surveys (15% of normal swine sera). Infection is apparently correlated with clinical problems in some cases; however, the true prevalence of clinical disease is difficult to determine.

B. Some serovars are adapted to other species and may incidentally infect swine.
   1. *L. icterohaemorrhagiae*—probably transmitted by rats.
   2. *L. canicola*—probably transmitted by dogs.
   3. *L. grippotyphosa*—probably transmitted by wildlife, including opossums, raccoons, muskrats, squirrels.
   4. *L. hardjo*—associated with cattle; infection of swine is unusual.

C. Organisms are transmitted through the urine of infected swine or other animal carriers (cattle, rats, dogs, wildlife, etc.).

D. May also be transmitted venereally.

PATHOGENESIS:

Organisms enter body through breaks in skin, mucous membrane, or conjunctiva → multiply in the blood stream → localize in the renal tubules and, in pregnant females, placenta and fetuses → organism may survive up to two years in the kidney and be chronically shed in the urine.

CLINICAL SIGNS:

A. Signs of illness in adult animals are mild and often go unnoticed.
   1. Anorexia
   2. Pyrexia
   3. Diarrhea
B. Abortions of late pregnancies (usually last trimester)
C. Stillborn and weak pigs
D. *L. bratislava* may be associated more with infertility than with abortion.

DIAGNOSIS:

A. Clinical signs are not specific enough for definitive diagnosis.
B. Culture
   1. Can be quite difficult.
   2. Is not routinely used for clinical diagnosis.
C. Dark-field microscopy—visualization of leptospires
   1. Of urine
   2. Of fetal fluids
D. Fluorescent antibody
E. Serology: must be interpreted in light of vaccination status.
   1. More useful as a herd test than as an individual animal test.
   2. Vaccination titers are usually 1:100 or less and persist only 3-6 weeks, while infection titers are usually 1:800 or greater.

TREATMENT AND CONTROL:

A. Vaccination
   1. Leptospira bacterins are widely used and generally effective at reducing losses from leptospirosis.
   2. Immunity from bacterins is relatively short-lived. Gilts should be vaccinated twice before the first breeding and sows should be vaccinated at or around every breeding (approximately every 6 months).
B. Treatment. Medication of feed with 400 g/ton chlortetracycline will help control clinical signs.

POSTPARTURIENT DYSGALACTIA

DEFINITION: A syndrome characterized by milk production by the sow insufficient to optimally maintain a litter of pigs.

SYNONYMS AND RELATED SYNDROMES:

A. MMA—mastitis, metritis, and agalactia
B. Agalactia toxemia
C. Lactation failure
D. Hypogalactia

ETIOLOGY:

A. Intramammary infections, e.g., *E. coli*, *Klebsiella*
B. Postpartum intrauterine infections, while theoretically capable of causing dysgalactia, are extremely rare in practice. Postpartum vaginal discharges do *not* usually indicate metritis.
C. Management problems
   1. Overfeeding or underfeeding
   2. Changes in feed
   3. Low fiber feeds
   4. Lack of exercise

   All of the above may lead to gut stasis and constipation.
D. Stress: thermal and other stresses
E. Toxins
   1. Ergot—more common if small grains (rye, barley, wheat) are fed.
   2. Aflatoxin
   3. Zearalenone
F. Nutrition: Vitamin E and selenium deficiency may predispose sows to dysgalactia.
G. Heredity
   1. Hypothyroid
   2. Hyperadrenal
   3. Basic ability to milk; especially colored breeds
H. Physical damage to teats, e.g., caught in slats or wire flooring, stepped on, etc.
I. Hysteria in sows (savage sow syndrome)

EPIDEMIOLOGY:

A. Average incidence of 7% to 17% is reported. May be higher or lower in an individual herd.
B. Incidence increases with the parity of the sow.
C. Infectious dysgalactia (classic MMA) may be greater in wet, unsanitary environments.

PATHOGENESIS:

A. Endotoxin mediated

   Gram negative bacterial infections (of any tissue but commonly the udder) or gastrointestinal stasis (constipation) can lead to systemic absorption of endotoxin. This can cause fever and anorexia in sow. Endotoxin also suppresses the release of prolactin and results in agalactia or hypogalactia.

B. Stress mediated—epinephrine and cortisol block action of oxytocin on myoepithelium.

C. Toxin mediated
   1. Ergot suppresses release of prolactin.
   2. Aflatoxin—unknown mechanism
   3. Zearalenone—estrogenic

CLINICAL SIGNS:

A. Endotoxin mediated
   1. Often occurs within the first 2-3 days following parturition.
   2. Sows may show:
      a. Depression
      b. Anorexia
      c. Pyrexia
      d. Constipation
      e. Enlarged, warm, discolored, sensitive mammary glands
   3. Pigs may show signs reflective of inadequate milk flow.
      a. Restless nursing behavior
      b. Slow growth
      c. Diarrhea (due to decreased flow of passive antibodies and subsequent enteric infection)

B. Other mediators
   1. May occur at any time during lactation.
   2. May see no clinical signs in the sow.
   3. Pigs show signs listed above in A.3.

DIAGNOSIS: May be difficult to get an etiologic diagnosis.

A. Clinical signs
B. Culture of inflamed mammary glands
C. Feed analysis for mycotoxins
D. Response to therapy or changes in management

TREATMENT: According to cause

(1-2ml)

A. Oxytocin: 30-50 units every 3 to 4 hours or as needed.

B. Antibiotics
   1. According to sensitivity
   2. Broad or Gram negative spectrum

C. Anti-inflammatory drugs
   1. Flunixin (Banamine)

Penicillin
Tylosin
Dypyrone
Acepromazine

milk + Karo syrup

Tx piglets also: for hypoglycemia not I.V.

a. Reduces fever and inflammation, may block effects of endotoxin.
b. Not approved for swine, extra-label use.

2. Corticosteroids
   a. Use is controversial.
   b. Should cover with antibiotics.

D. Tranquilizers
   1. Besides calming the hysterical sow, they may have direct lactogenic effects.
   2. Chlorpromazine is probably most effective at increasing release of prolactin; acepromazine or azaperone may also help.

E. Appetite stimulants for sow
   1. B vitamins
   2. Dog food
   3. Beer

PREVENTION AND CONTROL:

A. Clean and sanitary environment
B. Adequate water and laxative feed at and immediately prior to farrowing
C. Reduce environmental stress
D. Adequate exercise during the periparturient period
E. Anti-endotoxin vaccination (ENDOVAC-Porci, IMMVAC, Inc.)
F. Genetic selection for good milking sows

VULVAR DISCHARGE

ETIOLOGY:

A. Vulvar discharge may be associated with infection/inflammation of the urinary tract, uterus, or vagina.
   1. The most common isolates from the urinary tract are *E. coli*, *Proteus*, and *Eubacterium (Corynebacterium) suis*. In the southeastern United States, the kidney worm (*Stephanurus dentatus*) is also associated with urinary tract inflammation and discharge.
   2. The most common isolates from the uterus and vagina are *E. coli*, alpha and beta *Streptococcus*, *Proteus*, *Staphylococcus aureus*, and *Actinomyces (Corynebacterium) pyogenes*.

B. It is not known which if any of these organisms are primary pathogens. Most are likely opportunists.
C. Mixed infections are common.

PATHOGENESIS:

A. Little is definitively known.
B. Many of these bacteria are normally present in the vagina. Numbers of bacteria decrease from the caudal to cranial vagina.
C. Environmental bacteria may be introduced during breeding or during manually assisted farrowing.
D. The open cervix at estrus may allow organisms to ascend to the uterus.

CLINICAL SIGNS:

A. Urinary tract infection
    1. Amount of discharge is modest, usually < 20 ml.
    2. Discharge is usually seen during the final phases of urination.
    3. Discharge is usually unrelated to estrous cycle or reproductive status.
    4. Usually not associated with endometritis and infertility.
    5. Usually no systemic signs of illness.
B. Uterine infection—endometritis
    1. Amount of discharge is copious, often >100 ml.
    2. Discharge is usually seen within 6 days before estrus.
    3. Usually is associated with temporary or permanent infertility.
    4. Is more common in higher parity sows.
    5. Often there are no systemic signs of illness.
    6. May be associated with unsanitary breeding practices; however, even virgin gilts may develop endometritis.
    7. A moderate volume of discharge up to 3 days post farrowing may be considered normal. It is usually not associated with endometritis.
C. Vaginitis
    1. Amount of discharge is moderate, up to 50 ml.
    2. Discharge is unrelated to estrous cycle.
    3. Usually not associated with infertility unless infection ascends to the uterus.
    4. More common in gilts

Characteristics of the discharge are usually not of diagnostic value. Discharges are usually purulent and may be bloody. Mucoid discharges may be more common in urinary tract infections.

DIAGNOSIS:

A. May be difficult without postmortem examinations.
B. The most important diagnostic challenge is to determine whether discharges are affecting fertility.
    1. Analysis of reproductive records for evidence of increased levels of repeat breeding, anestrus, or failure to farrow.

2. Mechanical pregnancy diagnosis. Be aware, however, that a fluid-filled uterus may be falsely diagnosed as pregnant by A-mode ultrasound devices.

TREATMENT:

A. Treatment results are, at best, inconsistent. In most cases, if the discharge is determined to be affecting fertility, the animal should be culled.
B. If you must treat, choose an antibiotic based on culture and sensitivity. Some logical choices include tetracycline, potentiated sulfonamide, or aminoglycoside. Parenteral treatment is preferred. Intrauterine infusion of the sow is impractical due to the length and folds of the cervix. Feed antibiotics may not reach MIC levels.

PREVENTION AND CONTROL:

At this time, prevention and control measures are highly empirical and based on a sketchy understanding of the problem.

A. Cull all discharging sows that return to estrus or are nonpregnant by mechanical diagnosis.
B. Mate each sow to one boar only.
C. Use clean boars, not associated with discharging sows, on young sows and gilts.
D. Consider treating all boars and sows with long-acting tetracycline. Infusion into the sheath of boars may be useful in controlling infections.
E. Institute a mandatory clean-up of the entire breeding and early gestation area each week.
F. Cull sows after 6 or 7 litters. Old sows seem more prone to the problem.
G. Increase lactation length as much as possible to allow sows more time to clear up postparturient infections.
H. Review the hand mating procedure. If the manager is assisting the boar, insist on the use of clean gloves.

Suggested Reading:

Dial GD, MacLachlan NJ. 1988. Urogenital infections of swine. Part I. Clinical manifestations and pathogenesis. *Compend Contin Educ Pract Vet* 10: 63-71.

Dial GD, MacLachlan NJ. 1988. Urogenital infections of swine. Part II. Pathology and medical management. *Compend Contin Educ Pract Vet* 10: 529-540.

CYSTITIS/PYELONEPHRITIS

ETIOLOGY:

A. The most common cause of cystitis and/or pyelonephritis is *Eubacterium (Corynebacterium) suis*.
B. Several fecal or environmental organisms may opportunistically cause urinary tract infection (UTI); e.g., *E. coli*, *Klebsiella*, streptococci.

EPIDEMIOLOGY:

A. Sows are more commonly affected by UTI than are boars, barrows, and gilts. Pyelonephritis can be a significant cause of sow mortality.
B. Housing systems that limit activity and exercise (e.g., crates, tethers) may increase the risk of UTI. This is probably because crated or tethered sows drink less water and urinate less frequently than do group-housed sows.
C. Poor sanitation in the breeding and gestation areas of the farm may increase the risk of UTI.
D. Boars normally carry *Eubacterium suis* in their preputial diverticulum. This organism can be easily transferred to the sow at breeding.

PATHOGENESIS:

A. Bacterial organisms gain entry to the vagina during breeding or from fecal contamination of the perineal area. Under some conditions, these organisms establish an ascending urinary tract infection. Why some exposures result in infection and others do not is unclear.
B. *Eubacterium suis* has virulence factors that facilitate its ability to infect the urinary tract.
   1. It possesses pili, which mediate adherence to the bladder mucosa.
   2. It resists some of the natural urinary defense mechanisms. It does not react with Tamm Horsfall mucoprotein, which normally helps prevent bacterial adhesion to the mucosa of the urinary tract.
   3. It produces urease.
      a. Urease splits urea into ammonia, thus increasing the pH of the urine.
      b. *Eubacterium suis* grows best in an alkaline environment.
      c. Alkaline urine enhances the precipitation of struvite crystals, which may irritate the bladder and provide a matrix for bacterial growth.

CLINICAL SIGNS:

A. Early signs may include pyrexia, anorexia, and the observation of blood or pus in the urine.

B. Renal failure from pyelonephritis may result in polyuria/polydypsia, weight loss, and anorexia. Some cases result in sudden death with few observed clinical signs.

DIAGNOSIS:

A. Clinical pathology
   1. Urine pH is a useful clinical diagnostic procedure. Normal urine pH is 5.5 to 7.5, while a urine pH of 8 to 9 strongly suggests urinary tract infection. Plain pH paper is adequate for this measurement.
   2. Urinalysis may reveal blood, inflammatory cells, casts, and bacteria.
   3. Renal failure results in elevations of blood urea nitrogen and creatinine.

B. Postmortem pathology (necropsy or slaughter check)
   1. Urinary bladder may be hemorrhagic or necrotic and contain purulent material (cystitis).
   2. Ureters may be enlarged.
   3. Renal pelvis may contain a mixture of blood, pus, and urine. Microscopic exam may reveal inflammatory cells, bacteria, and casts in the renal tubules (pyelonephritis).

C. Culture: *Eubacterium suis* may be difficult to culture. Swabs should be placed in an anaerobic transport media (e.g., Kary Blair medium) and cultured anaerobically on selective media (e.g., colistin-nalidixic acid agar).

TREATMENT:

A. If diagnosed early, *E. suis* infection should respond to any of the penicillin family of antibiotics.

B. Ampicillin or amoxicillin have a broader antibacterial spectrum than penicillin G and may be preferable in treatment of UTI because of the possibility of coliform infections.

C. Urinary acidifiers (e.g., citric acid, vitamin C, D-L methionine, ammonium chloride) may be useful adjuncts to treatment.

D. If signs of renal failure are present, then prognosis for successful treatment is poor.

PREVENTION AND CONTROL:

A. Environmental hygiene. Keep the environment in the breeding and gestation areas clean. Remove manure from behind crated sows on a regular basis.

B. Breeding hygiene. Clean and disinfect breeding pens regularly. If assisting matings, use disposable gloves. Keep sow's perineal region clean during assisted matings.

C. Be sure that the sow has an adequate water supply.

D. Encourage activity in crated sows (e.g., frequent feedings, exercise time) as this will increase water intake and frequency of urination.

SEASONAL INFERTILITY

A. There is a seasonal drop in fertility for sows mated during the late summer months (July-September).

B. Almost all parameters related to reproductive performance are adversely affected—decreased conception rate, increased normal and delayed returns to estrus, increased weaning to first service interval. Decreases in conception rate of 10% to 15% are common in well managed herds during this time of year.

C. The cause is not entirely understood. Environmental temperature and/or photoperiod are presumed to be involved.

D. If the problem is severe, rule out other causes of infertility. Intensify efforts at good breeding management during these months (i.e., heat detection, multiple matings, increase energy intake to the sows prebreeding) and then accept the fact that this is going to happen and breed more sows/gilts in order to keep the farrowing crates full when November-January rolls around.

8

INTEGUMENTARY DISEASES

MANGE

ETIOLOGY: *Sarcoptes scabiei* var. *suis*

EPIDEMIOLOGY:

A. Mange infestation is extremely prevalent in U.S. swine herds.
B. Mite populations are greatest on chronically infected adult animals.
C. Mites are spread from animal to animal by direct contact, especially between a sow and her litter soon after farrowing.
D. Mites can survive for only a few days off the host. Low ambient temperatures enhance survival off the host.

PATHOGENESIS:

A. Mites burrow into the epidermis.
B. Females lay eggs in the epidermal tunnels.
C. Presence of mite may incite a hypersensitivity reaction resulting in pruritus.

CLINICAL SIGNS:

A. Acute allergic hypersensitivity
   1. Occurs most often in young nursery or grower pigs.
   2. Variable, but usually intense pruritus
   3. Papular dermatitis, especially on rump, flank, and ventral abdomen
   4. Lesions may progress to thickened, keratinized skin.
   5. Poor growth and/or feed conversion
      a. Most producers underestimate the negative economic effects of mange infestation.
      b. Mange infested pigs are probably more susceptible to other diseases

such as pneumonia and rhinitis.

6. Mites are usually *not* demonstrated on skin scrapings.

B. Chronic mange
   1. Usually occurs in adult breeding animals.
   2. Mild pruritus
   3. Thick, crusty scabs, especially in ear; occasionally around the head and neck
   4. Mites are usually present in large numbers and are easily demonstrated on skin scrapings.

DIAGNOSIS:

A. Clinical signs
B. Skin scrapings in chronic cases

TREATMENT AND CONTROL:

A. The transmission cycle of the mite can be broken by Caesarean delivery and isolation of pigs, therefore SPF pigs are free of mange.
B. Topical acaricides, e.g., sprays
   1. Several products are available. Examples include amitraz (Taktic—Hoechst), diazinon, fenvalerate, lindane, malathion, permethrin, phosmet (Prolate—StarBar).
   2. For severely infested swine, sprays should be applied 2-3 times at 14-day intervals (eggs are resistant to sprays but will have developed into susceptible adults by 14 days). For breeding animals, spraying should be repeated every 6 months.
   3. A common reason for inadequate mange control with sprays is inadequate application of the spray. The spray should be properly mixed and the animal thoroughly covered with the spray, especially in the ears.
C. Injectable acaricides, e.g., ivermectin
   1. Ivermectin (Ivomec—Merck) will kill 100% of adult mites with one injection at the recommended dosage (300 μg/kg—note the difference from the recommended cattle dosage of 200 μg/kg).
   2. Two injections of ivermectin 2 weeks apart to *every* animal in the herd will effectively eradicate mange from that herd.

LICE

ETIOLOGY: *Haematopinus suis*

EPIDEMIOLOGY:

A. The pig louse is very common, especially in poorly managed herds.
B. The pig louse is host-specific and cannot survive off the pig for more than 2-3 days.
C. Transmission is by direct contact with infested pigs.

PATHOGENESIS:

A. The louse lives, feeds, and reproduces on the surface of the pig's skin.
B. It pierces and sucks blood from the pig's skin, resulting in irritation and, in some cases, anemia.

CLINICAL SIGNS:

A. Pruritus
B. Anemia
C. Poor growth and feed conversion

DIAGNOSIS:

A. Pig lice are visible to the naked eye and often congregate about the neck, jowl, flank, and inside the ear.
B. Small white eggs (nits) can be seen attached to the hair.

TREATMENT AND CONTROL:

A. All of the treatments discussed for mange are also effective against lice.
B. Lousiness is relatively easier to control than mange.

EXUDATIVE EPIDERMITIS

SYNONYM: Greasy pig disease

ETIOLOGY: *Staphylococcus hyicus*

EPIDEMIOLOGY:

A. Usually affects pigs in the late preweaning to early postweaning stage.
B. Morbidity is usually low or moderate (up to 20%); mortality varies with age at onset and severity of signs (20% to 80%).
C. Poor environment and/or inadequate nutrition are sometimes associated with the disease.
D. The disease is sometimes seen after repopulation.

PATHOGENESIS:

A. Damage to the skin from external parasites (lice and mange), fighting, etc., may allow entry of the organism.
B. Certain strains of *Staph. hyicus* produce an exfoliative toxin that is believed to produce the characteristic skin lesions.
C. Pigs may die of dehydration and septicemia.

CLINICAL SIGNS:

A. Exfoliation of skin and excessive sebaceous secretion progresses to cracked, crusty skin that is covered with a brownish black malodorous exudate.
B. Listlessness, anorexia, and gauntness
C. Pyrexia and pruritus are *not* prominent clinical signs.

DIAGNOSIS:

A. Usually obvious from clinical signs.
B. Culture. Virulent and avirulent strains may be isolated from the same pig. This complicates interpretation of antimicrobial resistance tests.

TREATMENT:

A. Injectable antibiotics. Resistance to commonly used antibiotics (penicillin, oxytetracycline, lincomycin, erythromycin) is frequently encountered.
B. Prophylactic antibiotics in the feed, e.g., tetracycline
C. Clorox or Nolvasan dips
D. Antiseptic shampoos
E. Supportive care

PREVENTION AND CONTROL:

A. Improve environment: sanitation, ventilation, temperature.
B. Control external parasites.
C. Correct any nutritional deficiencies.

SWINE POX

ETIOLOGY: Swine pox virus

EPIDEMIOLOGY:

A. Once virus is established within a herd, it usually persists.
B. Outbreaks are sporadic; usually low morbidity and almost no mortality, especially in well-managed herds.
C. Poor sanitary conditions and lice infestation contribute to morbidity.
D. Generally affects only pigs less than 4 months of age.

PATHOGENESIS:

The virus enters through skin abrasions or via lice feeding. Replication occurs in the cytoplasm of skin epithelium. Regional lymph nodes may become reactive.

CLINICAL SIGNS:

A. Skin lesions progress through three stages:
   1. Papules: red, 1 to 6 mm in diameter
   2. Pustules: umbilicated, ischemic, yellow
   3. Crusts: brown to black
B. Progression of lesions occur over 1 to 3 weeks followed by complete recovery.

DIAGNOSIS:

A. Clinical signs
B. Skin biopsy: hydropic degeneration of cells in the stratum spinosum, intracytoplasmic inclusion bodies, central nuclear clearing

TREATMENT:

A. There is no specific treatment for swine pox nor is one really needed due to the innocuous effects of the disease.
B. Lice control is advised for herds with a lice problem.

9

CIRCULATORY DISEASES

MULBERRY HEART DISEASE

SYNONYM: Microangiopathy of pigs

ETIOLOGY: Vitamin E and/or selenium deficiency

EPIDEMIOLOGY:

A. Usually occurs in nursery or grower pigs but may occur at any age.
B. Feed grain processing (especially propionic acid treatment) may destroy vitamin E. Rancid fats may also destroy the vitamin.
C. Much of the lower Midwest has selenium-deficient soil. Cereal grains grown in these areas will be low in selenium.
D. Pigs may be better able to tolerate selenium deficiency if vitamin E is adequate than vitamin E deficiency if selenium is adequate.

PATHOGENESIS:

A. Vitamin E/selenium deficiency causes necrosis and failure of the myocardium.
B. Although the exact mechanism is not clearly understood, vitamin E and selenium are known to function as antioxidants. Presumably, lack of these nutrients increases the probability of oxidative damage to myocardial and endothelial cells.
C. Excess iron may enhance oxidative damage. Vitamin E and selenium seem to protect baby pigs from potential toxic effects of iron dextran injections.

CLINICAL SIGNS: Acute death

DIAGNOSIS:

A. Gross lesions
   1. Pericardial sac is filled with gelatinous fluid and fibrin.
   2. Myocardial and endocardial hemorrhage
   3. Hepatomegaly
B. Microscopic lesions: microthrombi in myocardial capillaries.
C. Hepatic selenium concentrations of less than 0.5 μg/g indicate selenium deficiency. A deficiency of vitamin E can cause also cause disease, therefore many cases will have normal levels of selenium.

TREATMENT AND CONTROL:

A. Vitamin E and/or selenium injections
B. Feed supplementation

BABY PIGLET ANEMIA

ETIOLOGY: Iron deficiency

PATHOGENESIS: The neonatal pig's iron requirement is greater than the sow's milk can provide. The pig can become significantly anemic within 2-3 days of birth.

CLINICAL SIGNS: Decreased growth rate, lethargy, pale skin and mucus membrane, dyspnea, edema, diarrhea

DIAGNOSIS:

A. Clinical signs
B. Hemoglobin < 6 g/100 ml (normal = 12-14 g/100 ml).

TREATMENT AND CONTROL:

A. Intramuscular injection of 200 mg iron in the form of iron dextran at 1 to 3 days of age is the treatment of choice. A second injection of iron 10 to 14 days later may be helpful in some herds.
B. Oral iron—inconsistent absorption

EPERYTHROZOONOSIS

ETIOLOGY: *Eperythrozoon suis* (rickettsia)

EPIDEMIOLOGY:

A. Infection has only been observed in domestic swine.
B. Serologic evidence of infection is more common than is clinical disease. Serologic infection rate of swine in the United States is 7% to 15%.
C. The disease is believed to be transmitted via blood-sucking arthropods (especially lice) and contaminated needles and surgical instruments.
D. Clinical expression of disease seems to be dependent on concurrent environmental, nutritional, or disease stress.

PATHOGENESIS:

Eperythrozoon suis is an obligate intracellular parasite of porcine erythrocytes. Acute clinical signs are due to intravascular hemolysis of parasitized erythrocytes. Experimental disease is difficult to reproduce except in splenectomized pigs.

CLINICAL SIGNS:

A. Acute disease
   1. Pyrexia
   2. Icterus and anemia
   3. Unthriftiness
   4. Acute disease is seen most often in nursing or recently weaned pigs.
B. Chronic disease
   1. Clinical signs are usually vague in infected adults.
   2. Chronic infection may have an adverse effect on reproductive performance, i.e., anestrus, decreased conception rate, abortion.

DIAGNOSIS:

A. Microscopic examination of blood smear
   1. Minute specks or rings within Giemsa stained erythrocytes
   2. Usually parasites can be detected only from acute, febrile cases.
B. Serology—indirect hemagglutination test
   1. Titers of 1:40 are considered suspect; 1:80 positive.
   2. Pigs less than 3 months of age rarely have titers.
   3. Only a few labs run this test.
   4. An ELISA has recently been developed.

TREATMENT AND CONTROL:

A. Oxytetracycline injected at 5 mg/lb or fed at 200 g/ton may control clinical signs but probably does not eliminate infection.
B. External parasite control, sanitation of surgical instruments

Index

Actinobacillus (*Haemophilus*) pleuropneumonia
  and mycoplasmal pneumonia, 49
  and pleuropneumonia, 45
Actinobacillus pleuropneumonia
  and swine influenza, 42
  vaccine for, 13
Actinomyces (*Corynebacterium*) *pyogenes*
  and foot lesions, 88
  and neonatal polyarthritis, 82
  and suppurative arthritis, 84
  vaccine for, 13
  and vulvar discharge, 100
Agalactia toxemia, 97–100
Air environment
  in disease management, 9
All in/all out rearing, 5–6
Ammonia control
  in air environment, 9
Anemia
  piglet, 112
AR. *See* Atrophic rhinitis (AR)
Arthritis
  mycoplasmal, 85–86
  suppurative, 84–85
Ascaris suum
  and verminous pneumonia, 51
Atrophic rhinitis (AR), 35–40
  vaccine for, 11–12
Aujeszky's disease (pseudorabies), 28–31
  vaccine for, 14

Baby pigs. *See* Piglets
Blue ear disease, 26–28
Bordetella bronchiseptica
  and atrophic rhinitis (AR), 35
  and bordetellosis, 43–44
  and segregated (medicated) early weaning (SEW, MEW), 7
  and streptococcal meningitis, 77
Bordetellosis, pulmonary, 43–44
Bowel syndrome
  hemorrhagic, 71–72
Bulbar paralysis
  infectious, 14, 28–31
Bullnose, 41

Campylobacter spp.
  and postweaning scours, 64
  and proliferative enteropathy, 70
Carbon monoxide
  in air environment, 9
Central nervous system diseases
  edema disease, 80–81
  myoclonia congenita, 75–76
  neonatal hypoglycemia, 76–77
  salt poisoning, 79
  streptococcal meningitis, 77–79
Circulatory diseases
  baby piglet anemia, 112
  eperythrozoonosis, 113–114
  mulberry heart disease, 111–112
Clostridial enteritis, 62–64
Clostridium perfringens type C
  and clostridial enteritis, 62, 63
  vaccine for, 13
Clostridium spp.
  and postweaning scours, 64
  and rotaviral enteritis, 60
CNS diseases. *See* Central nervous system diseases
Coccidiosis, 60–62
Colibacillosis, 5, 54–56
  vaccine for, 12
Congenital tremors, 75–76
Cystitis/pyelonephritis, 103–104

Dancing pig disease, 75–76
Depopulation/repopulation, 7
Discharge, vulvar, 100–102
Disease management
  by avoidance, 4–6
  by elimination, 6–7

Disease management (*continued*)
by environmental control, 8–10
by immunization, 10–14
by medication, 15–22
Dysentery, 66–69
vaccine for, 13

E. coli
and colibacillosis, 54–55
and edema disease, 80–81
and hemorrhagic bowel syndrome, 71
and postweaning scours, 66
and rotaviral enteritis, 60
and urinary tract infection, 103
vaccine for, 12
and vulvar discharge, 100
Edema disease, 80–81
EMC. *See* Encephalomyocarditis virus
Encephalomyocarditis virus
vaccine for, 14
Enteritis
rotaviral, 5, 13, 59–60
Enteropathy
proliferative, 70–71
Environmental control
in pathogen management, 8–10
Enzootic pneumonia, 85–86
Eperythrozoonosis, 113–114
Eperythrozoon suis
and eperythrozoonosis, 113
Epidermitis
exudative, 108–109
Erysipelas, 23–25
vaccine for, 11
Erysipelothrix rhusiopathiae
and erysipelas, 23
Escherichia coli. See *E. coli*
Eubacterium (*Corynebacterium*) *suis*
and cystitis/pyelonephritis, 103, 104
and vulvar discharge, 100
Exudative epidermitis, 108–109

Feces and urine, 9
Foot lesions, 88–89
Foot rot, 88–89
Fusobacterium necrophorum
and foot lesions, 88
and necrotic rhinitis, 41

Gastric ulcers, 73–74
Gastroenteritis, transmissible. *See* Transmissible gastroenteritis
Gastrointestinal diseases, 54–74
Glasser's disease, 5, 25–26
vaccine for, 13
Greasy pig disease, 108–109

Haematopinus suis
and lice, 108
Haemophilus parasuis
and atrophic rhinitis (AR), 35
and Glasser's disease, 25, 26
and porcine reproductive and respiratory syndrome (PRRS), 27
vaccine for, 13
Haemophilus pleuropneumonia
vaccine for, 13
Heart disease
mulberry, 111–112
Hemorrhagic bowel syndrome, 71–72
Herd management
in rearing, 5–6
in repopulation, 7
in size, 9–10
in SPF programs, 6–7
in weaning, 7
Hydrogen sulfide control
in air environment, 9
Hypogalactia, 97–100
Hypoglycemia
neonatal, 76–77

Ileobacter intracellularis
and proliferative enteropathy, 70, 71
Immunization
in pathogen management, 10–14
Inclusion body rhinitis, 40–41
Infectious bulbar paralysis (pseudorabies), 28–31
vaccine for, 14
Infertility
seasonal, 105
Influenza
swine, 14, 41–43
Integumentary diseases, 106–110
Isospora suis
and coccidiosis, 60

Lactation failure, 97–100
Laminitis, 88–89
Legs
splay-, 83–84
spraddle-, 83–84
Leptospira spp.
and leptospirosis, 96, 97
Leptospirosis, 96–97
vaccine for, 11
Lesions
foot, 88–89
Lice, 108

Mad itch (pseudorabies), 28–31
vaccine for, 14

Malignant hypothermia (MH), 92–93
Mange, 106–107
Mastitis, metritis, and agalactia (MMA), 97–100
Medicated early weaning (MEW), 7
Medication
  in pathogen management, 15–22
Meningitis
  streptococcal, 5, 77–79
Metastrongylus elongatus
  and verminous pneumonia, 51
MEW, 7
MH, 92–93
Microangiopathy of pigs, 111
Minimal disease herds, 6–7
Mulberry heart disease, 111
Multiple site production, 6
Musculoskeletal diseases, 82–93
Mycoplasma hyopneumoniae
  and mycoplasmal pneumonia, 48
  and segregated (medicated) early weaning (SEW, MEW), 7
  vaccine for, 14
Mycoplasma hyorhinis
  and mycoplasmal polyserositis, 44
Mycoplasma hyosynoviae
  and mycoplasmal arthritis, 85
Mycoplasmal arthritis, 85–86
Mycoplasmal pneumonia, 48–50
  vaccine for, 14
Mycoplasmal polyserositis, 44–45
Myoclonia congenita, 75–76
Myofibrillar hypoplasia, 83–84
Mystery pig disease, 26–28

Necrotic rhinitis, 41
Neonatal hypoglycemia, 76–77
Neonatal polyarthritis, 82–83

Osteochondrosis, 89–91
Osteomalacia, 91
Overcrowding, 4

Paralysis
  infectious bulbar, 14, 28–31
Parvovirus, 94–96
  vaccine for, 11–12
Pasteurellosis, 5, 50–51
Pasteurella spp.
  and atrophic rhinitis (AR), 11, 12, 35
  and pasteurellosis, 50–51
  and pneumonia, 47, 49
  and porcine reproductive and respiratory syndrome (PRRS), 27
Pathogen management
  by avoidance, 4–6
  by elimination, 6–7
  by environmental control, 8–10
  by immunization, 10–14
  by medication, 15–22
PEARS, 26–28
Piglets
  all in/all-out rearing, 5–6
  anemia, 112
  postweaning scours, 64–66
  splay-leg, 83–84
  weaning in disease control, 7
Pleuropneumonia, 45–48
  vaccine for, 13
Pneumonia
  mycoplasmal, 14, 48–50
  verminous, 51–53
Poisoning
  salt, 79–80
Polyarthritis
  neonatal, 82–83
Polyserositis
  mycoplasmal, 44–45
Polysystemic diseases, 23–34
Porcine epidemic abortion and respiratory syndrome (PEARS), 26–28
Porcine parvovirus, 94–96
  vaccine for, 11–12
Porcine reproductive and respiratory syndrome (PRRS), 26–28
Porcine stress syndrome (PSS), 92–93
Postparturient dysgalactia, 97–100
Postweaning scours, 64–66
Pox, swine, 110
Proliferative enteropathy, 70–71
Proliferative rhinitis, 41
Proteus
  and vulvar discharge, 100
PRRS, 26–28
Pseudorabies, 28–31
  vaccine for, 14
PSS, 92–93
Pulmonary bordetellosis, 43–44

Repopulation/depopulation, 7
Reproductive diseases
  porcine parvovirus (PPV), 94–96
  postparturient dysgalactia, 97–100
  seasonal infertility, 105
Respiratory diseases
  atrophic rhinitis (AR), 35–40
  inclusion body rhinitis, 40–41
  mycoplasmal pneumonia, 48–50
  mycoplasmal polyserositis, 44–45
  necrotic rhinitis, 41
  pasteurellosis, 50–51
  pleuropneumonia, 45–48
  pulmonary bordetellosis, 43–44
  swine influenza, 41–43

Respiratory diseases (*continued*)
  verminous pneumonia, 51–54
Rhinitis
  atrophic, 11–12, 35–40
  inclusion body, 40–41
  necrotic, 41
  proliferative, 41
Rickets, 87
Rotaviral enteritis, 5, 59–60
  vaccine for, 13

Salmonella spp.
  and pneumonia, 49
  and porcine reproductive and respiratory syndrome (PRRS), 27
  and postweaning scours, 64
  and salmonellosis, 43–34
  vaccine for, 14
Salmonellosis, 5, 32–34
  vaccine for, 14
Salt poisoning, 79–80
Sanitation
  in disease control, 5
Sarcoptes scabei var. *suis*
  and mange, 106
Scours
  postweaning, 64–66
Seasonal infertility, 105
Segregated early weaning (SEW), 7
Serpulina (*Treponema*) *hyodysenteriae*
  and postweaning scours, 64
  and swine dysentery, 66, 67, 69
  vaccine for, 13
SEW, 7
Shaker pigs, 75–76
SIRS, 26–28
Size of herd
  in disease management, 9–10
Social environment
  in disease management, 9–10
Sore feet, 88–89
Specific pathogen-free programs (SPF), 6–7
Splay-leg, 83–84
Spraddle-leg, 83–84
Staphylococcus spp.
  and exudative epidermitis, 108
  and vulvar discharge, 100
Stephanurus dentatus
  and vulvar discharge, 100
Streptococcal meningitis, 5, 77–79
Streptococcus spp.
  and neonatal polyarthritis, 82, 83
  and porcine reproductive and respiratory syndrome (PRRS), 27
  and streptococcal meningitis, 77
  and vulvar discharge, 100
Streptococcus suis
  and pneumonia, 49
  and streptococcal meningitis, 77, 78
  vaccine for, 13–14
Suppurative arthritis, 84–85
Swine infertility and respiratory syndrome (SIRS), 26–28
Swine influenza, 41–43
  vaccine for, 14
Swine pox, 110

Temperature control
  in disease management, 8–9
TGE. *See* Transmissible gastroenteritis
Thermal control
  in disease management, 8–9
Transmissible gastroenteritis, 56–59
  vaccine for, 12–13
Tremors
  congenital, 75–76
Treponema (*Serpulina hyodysenteriae*)
  vaccine for, 13
Trichuris suis
  and whipworms, 72, 73

Ulcers
  gastric, 73–74
Urine and feces
  ammonia from, 9
  hydrogen sulfide from, 9
Urogenital diseases
  cystitis/pyelonephritis, 103–104
  leptospirosis, 96–97
  vulvar discharge, 100–102

Vaccines. *See also* specific disease
  in pathogen management, 10–14
Verminous pneumonia, 51–53
Veterinarian's role
  in swine production, 3–4
Virus pig pneumonia, 85–86
Vulvar discharge, 100–102

Wastes
  ammonia from, 9
  hydrogen sulfide from, 9
Weaning
  in disease control, 7
  postweaning scours, 64–66
Whipworms, 72–73
Whooping cough, 43–44